True Nutrition

"Dr. March's new book explores the evolution of nutritional deficiencies in America and the subsequent deleterious impact on the health of our country. March's book is a historical review of changes to our food system and environment that have led to the ironic epidemic of diet-related health problems in the United States. This book is a valuable guide for anyone dealing with chronic illness who wants to optimize their health and is willing to use food as medicine."

Anne Kelly, M.D., M.P.H., FAAP, Founder, U Special Kids, University of Minnesota, Nutrition Ignition Inc. and the Nutrition Ignition Learning Lab

"If you read any book about the Mediterranean approach to healthy nutrition – this is the one to read!

It's fantastic. It'll set the record straight and tell you what you need for success."

Dr. Gary Epler, MD Boston Harvard Medical School Professor and Best-Selling Health Book Author

True Nutrition

European Secrets for American Women

Cocó March, ND

NEW YORK

True Nutrition
European Secrets for American Women

ISBN 978-1-61448-522-3 paperback
ISBN 978-1-61448-523-0 eBook
ISBN 978-1-61448-524-7 audio
Library of Congress Control Number: 2012955667

Morgan James Publishing
The Entrepreneurial Publisher
5 Penn Plaza, 23rd Floor,
New York City, New York 10001
(212) 655-5470 office • (516) 908-4496 fax
www.MorganJamesPublishing.com

Interior Design by:
Bonnie Bushman
bonnie@caboodlegraphics.com

In an effort to support local communities, raise awareness and funds, Morgan James Publishing donates a percentage of all book sales for the life of each book to Habitat for Humanity Peninsula and Greater Williamsburg.

Get involved today, visit
www.MorganJamesBuilds.com.

Habitat
for Humanity®
Peninsula and
Greater Williamsburg
Building Partner

Disclaimer

I wrote this book for informational purposes only. Any potential benefits discussed pertain to individual ingredients in the form of plants, not to the possible benefits of my dietary supplement formulas. Delicious Greens and Dr. Cocó Organic Greens, as well as all my other powder mixes, are dietary supplements. They are not intended to cure or treat diseases, or to replace the advice of your doctor. Information is power. What you do with that power is up to you.

When I state that a specific plant has been shown to have anti-cancer properties, for example, I am not making a claim about my product(s). I am simply sharing with you some of the findings published by independent researchers from universities and other institutions around the world. I do not make specific claims regarding the relative value or credibility of this evidence.

Scientists often spend years investigating the properties of specific phytonutrients. Many of these nutrients appear to possess beneficial properties, and that's why you should make sure you eat plenty of them daily. Not all the scientific evidence discussed herein can be considered equivalent. Some studies are preliminary, allowing no firm conclusions to be drawn yet. These statements have not been evaluated by the FDA. These products are not intended to diagnose, treat, cure, or prevent any disease.

For my son Marco, who died unexpectedly at age 2 from an accident; for his big brother Micah, who has taught me so much about life; and for my newborn son, Luca.

Dear Marco,

Mommy loved your eyes, daddy loved your smile, we both loved to hear your always cheerful laugh. We looked forward every morning to hold you in our arms, to kiss your cheek, to smell your hair. There was nothing we didn't love about you our dear Marco, nothing at all.

Your beautiful eyes are no longer open, but they soon will be, when Jesus calls your name and you wake up again.

We have a date our Marco Boy, we have a date in paradise that we won't miss for anything. We will be there with all those who love you so much, to hold you and kiss you while you grow up in a perfect new world where tears will be wiped away and death will be no more.

Love, Mommy and Daddy.

Table of Contents

Acknowledgments

The author wishes to acknowledge the following people who have helped make this book possible. Thanks to Dale Kiefer for his invaluable editorial advice, guidance and suggestions. Thank you John Cannell, M.D., Robert H. Lustig, M.D., and John McDougall, M.D., for allowing me to share tidbits of your wisdom in these pages.

To my support team, Betsy Dupre and Teng Thao, who kept me sane throughout the process of writing this book: Thanks for joining the Cocó March journey and helping me realize my dreams. This book would not have been possible without your priceless help.

I wanted to convey my appreciation to Dick Enrooth for challenging me more than a decade ago to be an entrepreneur. At the time, you didn't agree with my reason for pursuing success, but now you've joined in celebrating my accomplishments. I told you it would work! Thanks, too, to Linda Baggio for opening her home and for listening to my crazy ideas when I first arrived in America.

My gratitude to Zel Allen, author of "The Nut Gourmet," and "Vegan for the Holidays," for reviewing early drafts of the manuscript.

For his support, unconditional love, and kindness, I wish to thank the father of my children; my husband Mike.

Finally, I wish to thank the many individuals in my new homeland, the United States of America, who have treated me with patience, kindness and generosity since my arrival.

Introduction

There are so many things I love about America. I have been here for about fifteen years now, and this is my home. I was married here; my husband is American and my sons were born here. I love America's wide open spaces and friendly, open people. I've noticed and come to appreciate other things that most native-born Americans might not realize. One is the distinctly American attitude to things like customer service. We take it for granted that the customer is always right here, but to me this notion was an unexpected and welcome surprise. In most European countries they simply don't get it. Far from treating customers with utmost respect, in Europe customers are often made to feel as if they are a burden. Practically everyone in a service industry in Europe treats customers as if they are doing you a favor simply by doing their job.

I've also been touched by people's patience with me while I was still learning the language. I still recall how, during my first year here, my new friends would patiently explain things to me when I heard a new expression. They did this willingly, and without making me feel stupid, and I am grateful for their generosity.

I've also had occasion to experience people's kindness and support in time of need. Not very long ago, my youngest son, Marco, died in a tragic accident when he was just two years old. The pain of this horrible experience is still too raw for me to talk about, except to say that the kindness and love expressed by my community in suburban Minneapolis was an extraordinary comfort to my husband and me. Neighbors and friends brought food to us for weeks, a gesture that is not common in Europe. And I will never forget it.

I share this with you here because some of what I have to say may seem critical, and I don't want to sound like an outsider criticizing Americans and their habits.

The truth is that in America more than almost any other country you are continuously being exposed to an array of toxic substances found in ordinary places such as your food and water supply. Even less obvious sources of toxins include everyday items like cookware, shampoo and laundry detergent. On top of that, you are bombarded daily—minute-by-minute even—by marketing that promotes products as "healthy," when many of these products may actually be harmful. Or worse, lethal. While the products these companies promote may not be pure, their motives seem to be: This widespread deception is driven purely by the desire to make a buck.

This cycle needs to stop!

There's only one way. You need to take responsibility for your own health. Because no one else will. And that is why I wrote this book

If anything, my message is motivated by my love of my adopted country. I want to share my knowledge so that American women can live longer healthier lives. In the next few chapters, I'll present some of the data that supports why I advocate the need for a healthier you. Later chapters will provide easy-to-follow solutions to help you make simple dietary and lifestyle changes that can change your life.

I promise that by following my True Nutrition plan you can readily reinvigorate your energy, improve your digestion, achieve better and more restorative sleep, and sharpen your mental focus, among other improvements—while reaching your optimal weight. And all without the need for dieting. Best of all, my True Nutrition plan is a realistic approach to better health that's tailored to real-world American women and their families.

First, let me tell you how I made it to the land of plenty, the United States of America, and share with you the research that led me to create an easy-to-follow lifestyle plan.

PART I

Knowledge is Power

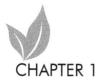

CHAPTER 1

The Shock

As I see it, every day you do one of two things:
build health or produce disease in yourself.
Adelle Davis

Like any young person heading off into the unknown, my emotions roiled between raw excitement and leaden trepidation. I was born in Germany; as the daughter of a Spanish father and a French mother, I had traveled extensively throughout Europe. I certainly didn't consider myself naïve or inexperienced. I possessed a newly minted degree as a naturopathic physician with a specialty in Nutrition, and a burning desire to further my understanding of the healing arts.

I was driven by a desire to broaden my education and expand my horizons, but my command of English was a bit tenuous. While being hosted by a loving American family with five beautiful children, I had arranged to continue my studies in the United States, at the University of Minnesota. The university is home to the world-renowned Mayo Clinic, and I had been attracted to the area by its sterling reputation as a bastion of medical innovation. I planned to augment my European doctor's degree by studying Food Science and Nutrition. Medicine runs through my veins, so to speak. My mother is a licensed practical nurse, while various cousins and uncles are M.D.s. I was proud to continue the family tradition. I was also motivated, in no small part, by the desire to improve my fluency in English.

Knowing no one, and tentative about the language, I was nevertheless fairly confident that I would confront the challenges ahead with aplomb. Then I stepped onto American soil, in northern Minnesota, in the dead of winter. In a raging snowstorm. The contrast with southern Spain, which I had so recently left behind, was shocking. Daunting, even. I was about to receive a far bigger shock, though—one that had far less to do with extremes in temperature, or the difficulties inherent in mastering a new language—and more to do with the often startling differences between cultures. In short, I was about to experience culture shock. I was in for some very big shocks indeed.

Cold, lonely, and feeling the anxiety of a stranger in a strange land, I stopped at a diner to get my bearings. Seeking warmth and comfort, I ordered a cup of coffee. When the waitress returned, I got my first surprise. The cup was enormous, far larger than the diminutive *demitasse* portion I was accustomed to receiving in Europe. I thanked the waitress and began nursing my coffee. I had scant money, and could afford little more than this solitary drink. Then came the second shock. The waitress soon returned with her steaming pot, and offered to refill my near-empty cup. "No, thank you," I replied, in my heavily accented English. She insisted. "Oh, no," I repeated, "I have had enough." In truth, I was worried about saving what little money I had left. I simply couldn't afford another cup of coffee. Soon she was back, again offering to refill my now empty cup. Again I refused, and again she insisted.

What I did not understand, and what she didn't know that I didn't know, was that she was offering free refills. *Free.* I was taken aback. In Europe, a second cup of coffee constitutes a second purchase. But here in the land of plenty, it seemed, some things are free.

Then I received my third shock of the day. As I looked around, I noticed something strange. Other patrons in the diner were ordering meals and eating them off enormous plates. I had to stop myself from staring, as staring is certainly considered rude behavior in any culture. But those plates! They were so enormous, I could scarcely believe my eyes. What's more, they were laden with equally enormous portions of food.

I also noticed that the only vegetable in sight was the occasional fried potato, dripping with grease, and a few lonely sprigs of parsley— evidently placed there as an afterthought. Indeed, the limp parsley appeared to be more of a decoration than a part of the cuisine. As a naturopathic physician with a special interest in nutrition (and having been raised vegetarian) I silently rued this emphasis on processed meats and empty carbs. Parsley is packed with powerhouse nutrients, and is used throughout the Mediterranean region as an integral ingredient in many cuisines and flavorful dishes. Far from being a neglected decoration, it is a prized ingredient that adds tang, color and brightness to many a dish.

As I continued to look about me, stealing surreptitious glances at other diner's leftovers, I noticed another unusual sight. People were paying their bills and departing the restaurant leaving mounds of food behind. A busboy cleared stacks of dishes, heaping them in a large bin as he struggled from table to table, clearing the remains of numerous uneaten portions of food. Not only are some things free, I noted, but food is so plentiful and cheap, people don't even bother to eat most of it. I soon realized I had a lot to learn about my new life in America.

That first glimpse of diners in the American heartland served as a sort of snapshot for me of all that is both wonderful and troubling about America's relationship with food. There is remarkable abundance; foods of every conceivable type and place of origin are readily available in massive supermarkets year-round. And much of this food is surprisingly affordable, but there is also rampant evidence of poor nutrition and outright malnutrition in this land of plenty. I've come to understand that this has less to do with the availability of nutritious food, and more to do with Americans' eating habits.

Food is so abundant we think nothing of leaving mounds of it behind on our plates. Portions are so large, we think nothing of piling it high on enormous plates that would be considered serving platters in much of Europe. There is so much emphasis on "meat and potatoes" that the bounty of nature in the form of fruits and vegetables often takes a backseat, or is ignored altogether, in favor of more meat (often processed beyond recognition) and more potatoes (usually deep fried and slathered with salt). As I witnessed that first bewildering day in the land of plenty, tokens from the plant kingdom are relegated to the edge of the plate, where they are neglected as disposable garnishes.

I received yet another shock on that frigid day in Minnesota. Although it hardly warrants notice these days, I was startled by the number of overweight and obese people packed into that diner. They were eating heaping plates of fried potatoes, enormous hamburgers, skyscrapers of pancakes dripping with artificial syrup and melted butter, entire rashers of greasy bacon and multi-egg omelets. In the following weeks, I would receive other surprises. I still recall writing letters to my friends back home in Barcelona, in which I breathlessly described the exotic practices I had recently witnessed. Coffee is occasionally served in paper cups (paper cups!), for drinking "on the run;" meals are served through little windows to people sitting in cars, who then drive away to "eat on the run." Families don't sit down to eat meals together routinely; some families *never* gather to share a meal, except at holidays, when the tables groan with more food than anyone can possibly eat in one sitting. Children drink sugary soft drinks— and nothing else—throughout the day.

Of course, at first, I was simply having trouble getting used to the idea of meals eaten in the car and drinks to go. Clearly I had a lot to learn about America, and America, I thought to myself, has a lot to learn about nutrition. It was then that I decided my mission was clear: We will learn from each other.

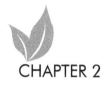

CHAPTER 2

Secret One: Take Charge

The first order of business of anyone who wants to enjoy success in all areas of his or her life is to take charge of the internal dialogue...and only think, say and behave in a manner consistent with the results they truly desire.
Sidney Madwed

When you think of women who changed the world, who comes to mind? Indira Gandhi, for her political achievements? Marie Curie, for being the first woman ever to win two Nobel Prizes? Or Margaret Thatcher, for being elected Prime Minister of the United Kingdom, for an unprecedented three consecutive terms?

Although we all admire the tenacity of these amazing women, I am sure most of you will agree that they did not directly affect your personal life. But what if I told you there is a way you can have an impact not just in your own life, but also on the lives of those around you, those who you love the most: your family and your friends?

I am a wife and a mother, and I am currently pregnant with my third child. If you read the Introduction, you know that my second son, Marco, died in an accident at age two. I certainly hope you have not lost any loved ones. Although the emptiness of his absence still keeps awake at night, I hope that some good may come of this tragedy. Losing Marco inspired me to write this book and share my knowledge with you.

Taking charge of your life is the most important thing you can do as a woman, especially if you are a mom like me. Your children will learn from your example, and they will pass on that learned behavior onto their own children, just like I am sure there are many things you do daily which you learned from your mom, hence the importance of taking charge.

CPR

Most people know that CPR is an emergency technique that saves lives. When a life hangs in the balance, it can be performed by anyone, anywhere, at any time. I've adopted this acronym for my True Nutrition mantra. Whether you are a mother or not, CPR is relevant to you. My True Nutrition plan is about taking charge of your life, and here's why: First, because you Can, second because you have the Power, and third because you have the Right. Repeat with me: I <u>Can</u>. I have the <u>Power</u>. I have the <u>Right</u> to take charge. That's my version of CPR. I want you to keep it in mind at all times, particularly if you choose to make changes to better yourself and someone asks "why"? Why do you want to change your lifestyle or eating habits or dress habits? Remember CPR.

By taking charge you will make changes. You may not be able to change the world. You may never be listed as one of the top one hundred women of the century (or perhaps you will, who knows?) But even so, what good does it do to save the world if you are unable save yourself?

Stopping the Cycle

I am here to help you take charge of your life and teach you the secrets that will lead to a happy, healthy you. If you purchased this book it is perhaps because you have heard me on the radio or watched me on TV, and you were inspired to do more than you have been doing; to do things differently than you've been taught.

This may mean unlearning some of the things you learned from your own mother. If you are a victim of any of the common diseases that have become so prevalent in the United States—conditions such as obesity (which I consider a disease in itself), or the trickle-down effect of being overweight, having high blood pressure, diabetes, high cholesterol, or heart disease to name a few—I know you can improve and even reverse many of these conditions simply by following my secrets.

In Europe, we say that America is considered number one in most areas. There is a bit of unspoken jealousy among Europeans. I know this because I am European. I was born in Germany. My mother is French and my father is from Spain. I have lived in several countries and traveled throughout Europe extensively. Although they will never say so, Europeans would like to enjoy some of the comforts and resources that America seems to have in abundance. To be honest, it's one of the reasons I stayed.

I agree that the United States of America is the land of opportunity. It is a nation that empowers individuals to succeed. Unfortunately, chronic diseases are another area where we're number one. Many health conditions that have set off alarm bells in this land of plenty have slowly spread throughout other parts of the world as those far flung places have adopted American habits. We certainly *don't* want to be number one at lifestyle diseases. It's up to you to stop the cycle, at least in your own family.

How True Nutrition Was Born

This is a plan I have been developing for decades. It is informed by my early years living in Europe, and by a strong tradition of healing in my family. It was strongly influenced by the experiences of my mother, a practical nurse who, by implementing its principles, miraculously overcame an illness that conventional physicians had labeled "intractable." It was forged during the years of my training as a doctor of naturopathy and further refined throughout my years of medical practice, where I gained real-world insight into the health challenges average Americans face every day.

It has been further honed by my experiences as a mother confronting her children's health challenges, as well as the challenges of patients that sought my counsel. The implementation of the principles you will find in this book was responsible for transforming the lives of many people.

I became a practitioner out of a deep-seated desire to help people heal and achieve wellness. In my practice I routinely treated patients with conditions ranging from diabetes to heart disease and cancer. I became convinced that most of these patients' problems could be traced back to their dietary and lifestyle habits over the previous ten to fifteen years of their lives. Invariably these patients came to me after years of ignoring advice to get regular exercise and eat a healthful diet.

The link between poor diet and conditions like obesity and cancer seemed obvious to me, and I was able to help many of these people reverse their diseases and take control of their lives by working with them to make better dietary choices, by helping them take charge of their lives.

By doing what you are doing right now, you have already taken the first tentative step toward sustainable wellness for yourself and your loved ones. In some regards, this is one of the easiest steps of all. It involves no actual action on your part; no sacrifice, expenditure, or pain. By reading this book, you've already shown that you are interested in improving your life and that you are in charge. And that's half the battle. The rest is details.

STEP ONE: Change your Mind

The first step is simply to change your mind. I can tell that you have already decided on some level that you are interested in better health. As the saying goes, you don't have to be sick to seek wellness. But you must acknowledge that there is room for improvement, before you can take action to bring about change.

Whether it means eating better, cooking fresher, buying organic, investing more time in family meals enjoyed together, learning to relax, or exercising more regularly, you've at least acknowledged that you're ready to make some changes for the better. For better health and, possibly, for a better life.

Of course, this is at once one of the simplest yet most challenging of all possible tasks. For to change one's mind is to initiate change in one's life; to summon change in the "real" world. Sounds simple enough, but make no mistake: Without changing the way you think—without embracing new ideas about everything from diet and exercise, to lifestyle—you cannot hope to implement real change in your life.

In medicine we are constantly confronted with the need to change. New studies, new information, new procedures, novel medications, unexpected or contrary findings—all of these require modern physicians and health care professionals to be flexible.

We must be willing not only to be open to new information, but to new ideas. We must work to monitor advances in the many interdisciplinary fields that contribute to medical knowledge, and be able to set aside old, obsolete ideas and adapt to this new knowledge, as our understanding of the human body and human disease changes.

Sometimes, what is old is new again. Much of the knowledge that informs naturopathic medicine derives from ancient wisdom. It is the wisdom of herbs, and plants, and the ancient dietary patterns and lifestyles of our ancestors.

It is informed by ancient systems of medicine that consider the whole patient in the context of his or her own life, rather than isolated symptoms and complaints. It seeks wellness through balance, and the removal of potential toxins (primarily of man-made origin), and a diet based on lean protein, whole grains, fruits, vegetables, nuts and seeds. It emphasizes the inherent ability of one's own body to heal itself and achieve harmony and wellness.

Unlike some—who may have heard of the benefits of a natural lifestyle and a whole-foods, plant-based diet, but have not seen the benefits of choosing it—I am always mindful of what my mother experienced. Some fifty years ago she was told by the medical community that she was going to die. Thankfully, she proved them wrong, and her personal story is living proof of the benefit of taking charge of you own life.

STEP TWO: Make Changes

If you believe in destiny you may trust that fate has dictated what the future holds for you. My mother's story showed me that rather than destiny, we are in charge of our own paths; that we create our future through the choices we make in the present. Her story taught me that if we believe strongly enough, we can change the outcome of many situations, because WE ARE IN CHARGE of our own decisions, and most things that affect our lives.

Mom is a licensed practical nurse. In her late twenties, while studying to become a medical doctor, Mom contracted hepatitis from an infected needle. She was so sick for so long that everyone thought she was going to die. She was in bed for several months. Eventually she was released from the hospital and sent home.

Her hepatitis seemed to be cured, but she was frail and sickly most of the time. To put it simply, Mom could neither function nor care for herself as she once did, and she was still so young. Her symptoms were attributed to her ailing liver, so she was prescribed endless medications to help her liver improve.

After years of struggling with low energy and a general lack of vitality, she decided to visit a different clinic, where they took a more holistic approach to medicine. By now she was desperate for alternative solutions to her liver problems, which seemed to worsen with each passing day. To her great surprise she received some additional alarming news: After everything she had endured, her liver was not in the best shape, but her liver was not the primary cause of her current problems. To her shock, she was told that an altogether different problem had developed.

She was diagnosed with chronic nephritis; a serious inflammation of the kidneys. Nephritis? Mom was beside herself. Nephritis is often caused by infections, toxins and autoimmune diseases. In Mom's case, the overload of toxins generated by the massive amounts of medications she had been prescribed to heal her liver from hepatitis had subsequently caused her kidneys to become inflamed. They were close to failing, and that can be fatal.

So now that she had conquered hepatitis, she was approaching her deathbed again. The only remaining option was dialysis. Dialysis artificially extracts toxins from the blood, doing the work of the kidneys by keeping potentially deadly poisons from building up in the bloodstream. It is a sort of living death sentence. It requires spending countless hours hooked up to a machine several times a week. Short of organ transplant or death, there is no going back once you start. As a healthcare professional, my mother was well aware that going on dialysis meant her quality of life would take a nosedive.

She was unwilling to give up hope and accept her fate. She stubbornly decided there simply had to be a better way. So she refused dialysis. She became her own health advocate and began investigating alternatives. In those days, the term "alternative and complementary medicine" was relatively unfamiliar. In my view, she was an early pioneer.

To take stress off her kidneys, Mom became a vegan. For those of you who may not know, veganism is a lifestyle that embraces foods solely from the plant kingdom, while rejecting the consumption of any animal products. While vegetarians may or may not eat some dairy products or eggs, vegans abstain from those foods.

In any event, my mother understood the benefits and potential shortcomings of veganism, and in her desperation she embraced this new diet wholeheartedly. She also delved deeper into natural therapies and traditional approaches to healing. Mom decided that no one was going to dictate her future any more. To Mom's surprise, after changing her lifestyle completely, she slowly began to regain her energy and health. Soon she was able to go back to her job as a Practical Nurse, while continuing her education to become a physician.

Becoming a pure vegan was the answer to my mom's critical condition. I am not a vegan now, although I was raised as one and didn't eat animal products until I was in my twenties. And I am not suggesting you should discontinue all meat consumption to regain your health. Rather, I believe that taking charge of your health may require different actions for different people according to their unique situations. In my mom's case, eliminating any food that could cause inflammation of her kidneys was her way to take charge and it worked.

Mom was just a few credits shy of earning her M.D. degree when she fell in love and married my father, and they subsequently moved to Germany, where my dad already lived. Mom had so much to live for. She was still a young woman, with a husband and a promising career. In the ensuing years, despite her health challenges, she had three healthy children. As a result of her experiences, we were raised as vegetarians. Today, fifty-odd years later, mom continues being a vegan, and is still well, despite being told she would die without dialysis.

And that demonstrates the amazing power of a whole-foods, plant-based diet. My mother played a tremendous role in my decision to study and practice nutrition and natural medicine, with an emphasis on food science, rather than pursue a career in conventional medicine.

What can you do to take charge of your health? Start with a positive dialogue that will create a productive mind set. Why? Because whether you want to lose weight, be more energetic, reduce or eliminate muscle and joint pain, eradicate mental fogginess, be more focused, or cure a chronic disease, the power and desire to do so starts in your mind.

Your mental dialogue is between you and yourself. You can't let any negativity come in between.

 ## Secrets to remember:

- You are your own boss
- You control your thoughts
- You are in charge of yourself
- This is the time to make changes
- Any positive change is worth making
- You don't need to make all changes at once
- Others have made it, YOU WILL MAKE IT!
- If a friend tells you that you can't do it, get rid of that friend

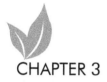

CHAPTER 3

Remove the Veil

Quit worrying about your health. It'll go away.
Robert Orben

Health is not valued till sickness comes.
Dr. Thomas Fuller

*The doctor of the future will no longer treat the human frame with drugs,
but rather will cure and prevent disease with nutrition.*
Thomas Edison

D eath. It's the great equalizer. Rich, poor, black, white, tall, short; no matter who you are or where you came from, you can't escape the simple fact that we all die eventually. Despite this inescapable reality, people have always longed for, even strived for, eternal life. For centuries, practitioners of alchemy pursued the elixir of life, a mythical potion that was purported to grant the drinker eternal, youthful life.

Diverse cultures from China to India to Europe have all searched for this imaginary concoction. The most famous Chinese alchemical book, the Tan Chin Yao Ch'eh ("Great Secrets of Alchemy"), dating from approximately 650 AD, discusses the creation of elixirs for immortality in detail.

The ingredients for this miraculous potion were a concoction of metallic elements and salts, including mercury, sulfur, and arsenic. Of course, modern readers will realize that, rather than contribute to longevity, many of these substances are acutely toxic.

Jiajing Emperor, of the Ming Dynasty, died from ingesting a lethal dose of mercury in the alleged "Elixir of Life" conjured by his court alchemists. Historians are confident that many other emperors died at the hands of so-called alchemists proffering "magical" potions.

Of course, it is now the twenty-first century and information is readily available at our fingertips. We know there is no Elixir of Life and that ancient potions claiming to confer eternal life were actually foul poisons. But the desire for longer life never goes out of style. We still want to extend our lifespans, and with today's technology we should be doing so. But are we living longer, or are we just being quietly killed?

The Facts of Life and Death in America

In an opinion piece published in the influential medical journal, *Circulation*, in early 2011, the editorial board of the American Heart Association announced that costs due to heart disease—our most common killer—will skyrocket by 2030 to more than $800 billion per year. Remarkably, the United States has the highest expenditures for health care of any nation on the planet.

The authors of this sobering projection concluded their report by warning "effective prevention strategies are needed" to rein in the burgeoning burden of heart disease. If implemented, well-established "prevention activities" (many of which we will discuss in this book) could reduce the incidence of heart attacks and strokes by about two-thirds and one-third, respectively, the AHA estimates.

This book is about taking responsibility for—and control of—your health and the health of your loved ones. Some of the steps may be easier than others, but given the costs of inaction, you've got to ask yourself: Can I afford *not* to take action?

Reject the notion of victimhood. If you are one of the millions of Americans with pre-diabetes, or full-blown type 2 diabetes, you may believe you have been afflicted by a cruel and inevitable condition. Drugs in rising doses are your future now, you are told. You're another victim of diabetes in modern America.

Wrong.

Diabetes is cruel, but it's not unavoidable. Reject the notion of victimhood. You are only a victim if you believe you are. Diabetes is entirely preventable, ditto heart disease, with very few exceptions. These and other rampant conditions—obesity, hypertension, kidney disease, the metabolic syndrome—are all preventable.

If any of these conditions have already been diagnosed, they can be controlled through natural means. In many cases, these conditions can be improved, or even reversed through natural approaches. It all starts with a change of mind. It begins when you reject victimhood and take responsibility for loving yourself and your family enough to eat right and stay fit. Diabetes is not inevitable. The nation's number one killer, heart disease, needn't claim you.

Lifestyle

America is a global leader in many diseases. Unfortunately, there is much about Americans' diets and lifestyles that contributes to disease, rather than wellness. This is distressing to me because I know that an excellent diet can be the source of excellent health. Many factors are involved in this dysfunctional relationship with food, but they can be boiled down to this: The typical American eats too many calorie-dense foods and too few nutrient-dense foods. Calorie-dense foods are high in calories, often from fats or sugars, but they're low in nutrients, such as fiber, vitamins, minerals and, perhaps most importantly, phytonutrients (nutrient compounds from plant sources).

Calorie-dense foods are high in calories and, of course, excess calories contribute to weight gain. Oceans of ink have already been spilled describing the problems posed by rampant obesity, so I won't belabor the issue here. Suffice it to say that obesity is epidemic in this and other developed countries, and it's even showing up in young children at unprecedented rates. Just recently, the results of yet another study were published, showing that children who are obese are at dramatically higher risk of suffering from heart disease than their normal-weight peers.

An Ounce of Prevention is Worth a Pound of Cure

Obesity is associated with greater incidences of a host of diseases and conditions, ranging from cardiovascular disease (still the *number one* cause of death in both men and women in America), to type 2 diabetes, high blood pressure, sexual dysfunction, kidney disease, arthritis and even cancer. When several of these conditions coexist, we usually speak of the metabolic syndrome; an affliction that is shockingly common today. The metabolic syndrome is characterized by a combination of three or more of the above conditions, and represents an appallingly poor state of health and an alarmingly high risk of disability and death.

The single common thread among all these diseases and the metabolic syndrome is invariably obesity. Sadly, these so-called "lifestyle" diseases are largely preventable. Yet American medicine—to the tune of billions of dollars every year—is almost exclusively focused on *reactive*, rather than *preventive*, medicine.

Conventional medicine, especially in this country, is far more likely to treat a disease after it manifests, rather than encouraging steps to prevent it from occurring in the first place. Prevention starts with a good diet, and statistics suggest that in America we're paying an exorbitantly high price for our addiction to unhealthful foods and sugar-laden drinks.

Unfortunately, emerging science suggests that some foods may be truly addictive. This may sound silly. It's a little like saying air is addictive. But the thinking behind this idea merits consideration. If certain types of foods are more likely than others to trigger hunger, or the deposition of fat, it might well be possible to use this knowledge to tame our appetites and help us shed unwanted pounds.

Would you like to guess which foods have been identified as acting like addictive substances? If you guessed "anything with sugar and fat" (cupcakes anyone?), you're right. According to preliminary (but mounting) evidence, foods laden with sugar and fat are not *inherently* addictive, but they are capable of triggering certain changes in the brain that, over time, result in these foods *becoming* effectively addictive. In this scenario, sugary/fatty foods provoke a cycle of abstinence and binging. And this pattern of eating has been associated with obesity, early weight gain, depression, and even anxiety.

Beyond Mere Color

Calorie-dense foods also tend to be highly processed. In contrast to whole, fresh foods—which come to us directly from nature, much as God intended—processed foods are subjected to any number of industrial processes. These processes often involve the removal of beneficial nutrients (such as fiber and phytonutrients), while simultaneously adding artificial ingredients of questionable virtue, such as chemical preservatives, food colorings, flavor "enhancers," fillers, etc.

Food dyes are only the latest example of chemicals permeating our modern food supply that have garnered notoriety in the media recently. A number of studies have concluded that these artificial chemicals are implicated in hyperactivity disorders among susceptible children. Despite having been approved for human consumption for decades, these dyes have been shown to play an important role in triggering, or worsening, symptoms of hyperactivity among certain children. In early 2011, the United States Food and Drug Administration announced that it would hold hearings on the matter. I'm tempted to suggest that this may be too little, too late.

Hyperactivity disorders, including Attention Deficit Disorder (ADD) and Attention Deficit Hyperactivity Disorder (ADHD), are alarmingly common in this country. How has this startling increase in children with ADD and ADHD been addressed? Scores of children are currently taking potent medications on a daily basis to treat the symptoms of these conditions.

Some of you may be old enough to recall a time when certain food colorings were suddenly declared unsafe and were removed from the market. Does anyone remember Red Dye Number 2? It was forced out of the food supply after its consumption was linked to an elevated risk of cancer in laboratory rodents. Even less well known is the fact that artificial food dyes may contain traces of the organic solvents that are used in their manufacture. This includes known toxins such as acetone and hexane. In pure form, these solvents are suspected carcinogens. In Europe, certain dyes are not recommended for consumption by children and in certain European countries they are already banned outright. Meanwhile, in the United States they are still used by the manufacturers of many foods.

MSG

Another common additive in prepared foods (particularly savory snack foods, like chips and crackers) is the "flavor enhancer" monosodium glutamate (MSG). Food scientists, those industrial folks who "design" foods for mass production and consumption, realized long ago that by adding MSG to processed foods they could cheaply enhance consumers' perceptions about the irresistible savoriness of a given product. For this reason, MSG is now featured in a wide range of products.

Occasionally listed under varying terms, ranging from "autolyzed protein extract" to "hydrolyzed yeast extract," manufacturers have made it difficult for wary consumers to detect—and thus avoid—this additive in their food products. Some have suggested that its effects are addictive, promoting excessive eating. This claim remains controversial, however. Various studies have reported conflicting findings regarding MSG's effects on weight gain.

MSG provides a taste quality called "umami;" one of the five basic tastes, along with bitter, sour, salty and sweet. Borrowed from the Japanese language, *umami* describes a quality that is often referred to as savoriness. It is sometimes also described as brothy, or meaty. Specific taste receptors react to the presence of an amino acid, glutamic acid, or more specifically, to glutamate salts. MSG is one of these.

Problem is, MSG may have undesirable effects on appetite. Although research on the subject remains inconclusive, it has been suggested that some individuals are sensitive to MSG, and may suffer some side effects related to its consumption. Other research has suggested that it interferes with the body's normal *satiety circuit*; the complex system of feedback loops, mediated by various hormones and sensory structures, which tells us when we are hungry and when we are full. One is left to wonder what purpose this additive serves, beyond enticing us to eat more of prepared snack foods that often provide empty calories and excess salt, and little in the way of nutrition.

Innocent Snacks

The average American will eat potato chips more than occasionally. You may think of chips as a harmless snack, but this calorie-dense food also tends to be highly processed. This processing includes cooking food to the point that it becomes essentially worthless from a nutrition standpoint, and potentially dangerous to your health.

Potatoes are an inexpensive source of energy, and potatoes have been comfort food for many centuries. However, when potatoes—or any starchy food—are deep fried at high temperatures a toxic compound is formed. This byproduct of high-temperature cooking is called acrylamide. When these foods are cooked at lower temperatures (by boiling, for example) these toxic compounds are not formed. Unfortunately, french fries and potato chips are packed with acrylamides. In fact, the deeper "golden brown" these foods are, the higher their levels of acrylamides are likely to be.

Acrylamides

Acrylamides are suspected of causing cancer. In fact, a large Dutch study completed in 2009 showed that people with the highest dietary intake of acrylamides (or people who consumed the largest amounts of chips and deep fried carbohydrate foods, like donuts) were 59% more likely to develop cancer of the kidneys.

Cancer is not the only problem caused by deep fried foods or foods that contain nasty acrylamides. According to the results of a study published in the *American Journal of Clinical Nutrition*, eating plenty of fried foods, such as potato chips, can dramatically increase inflammation. Inflammation is now known to play a role in the development of many of the illnesses that are so common in the United States today, including arthritis, Alzheimer's disease, heart disease, and—not surprisingly—cancer. Atherosclerosis, for example, is the root cause of most cardiovascular disease. And atherosclerosis is now recognized as an inflammatory condition.

After all this information you may wonder, how many chips can I eat before they are harmful?

The *Journal of Clinical Nutrition* study showed that consumption of just six ounces of potato chips daily, for one month, results in significantly increased levels of oxidized LDL-cholesterol in the blood stream. When LDL cholesterol is oxidized it becomes harmful, which is why it's often referred to as "bad cholesterol."

This illustrates some of the hidden dangers of mindlessly snacking on "junk food." I suspect that most people think of these kinds of foods as bad for them because they are so high in fat, carbs and calories. But sometimes processed foods have a negative effect on health that goes deeper than just empty calories, or even excessive amounts of salt.

"You can't change other people, but you can change yourself" is an accurate statement. You have the power to makes changes within yourself. I believe that even small changes dramatically impact your health. Good or bad, big or small, the choices you make every day affect your health and your life. To change the way you act and feel, you have to change the way you think.

 ## Secrets to remember:

Start with small changes. You don't have to go conquer the whole world right away to notice changes in your body. Start by doing the following:

- Read labels. If a product contains MSG, which can also be listed as yeast extract, anything "hydrolyzed," hydrolyzed protein, calcium caseinate, sodium caseinate, yeast food, yeast nutrient, or autolyzed yeast, do not buy it. Go through your kitchen cabinets. If you see this ingredient in your food, toss it. I know it's hard, but why poison yourself?

- Avoid food colorants; they will adversely affect your brain chemistry. Like MSG they have been linked to behavioral problems.

- Snacking is great, but don't snack on chips. Replace them with nuts, Greek yogurt, or plain fruit.

- Go to my website and download my free report. Enter the search terms "hidden MSG" at CocoMarch.com.

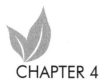

CHAPTER 4

Invisible Killers—
Things Keeping Your
Fat from Saying Goodbye

Sweet, sweet, sweet poison for the age's tooth.
William Shakespeare

I n April 2010, the online version of *Time* magazine published an article entitled "Top 10 Common Household Toxins: The Hazards Lurking at Home." The article listed an alarming collection of harmful chemicals, many of which are common in most American homes. The list of potentially hazardous chemicals included everything from chemicals used in cosmetics, to synthetic preservatives, to common sunscreen ingredients, to additives in lip balm, hair care and shaving products.

Even children's toys harbor phthalates. These are potentially harmful, widely distributed chemicals that are added to many plastics to provide resilience and flexibility. This class of chemicals has been linked to human liver cancer, reduced sperm counts, and other reproductive abnormalities. Numerous other common chemicals also act as endocrine disruptors, interfering with the normal activity of hormones ranging from thyroid hormones to estrogens.

Unfortunately, living a life free of toxins is discouragingly difficult in the twenty-first century. Studies have repeatedly reported that a stew of troubling chemicals circulates in the bloodstreams of ordinary Americans. This widespread contamination includes a broad range of toxins, ranging from heavy metals, such as mercury and lead, to endocrine disruptors, and virtually indestructible substances called perfluorochemicals.

In early 2011, the troubling issue of environmental toxins—ranging from bisphenol A (BPA) in food packaging and phthalates in flexible plastics, to triclosan in soaps and PBDE flame retardants in furniture and other products—prompted the American Academy of Pediatricians to issue a new policy statement, aimed at encouraging the federal government to overhaul the provisions of the Toxic Substances Control Act of 1976.

The Act empowers the Environmental Protection Agency (EPA) to monitor, test and regulate or restrict certain chemicals. Excluded are foods, drugs and pesticides, which are ostensibly regulated by the United States Food and Drug Administration (FDA).

The academy's statement reads, in part: "[The Toxic Substances Control Act] is widely recognized to have been ineffective in protecting children, pregnant women, and the general population from hazardous chemicals in the marketplace." The statement goes on to admonish EPA, noting that in the 35-year history of the act, only five chemicals or chemical classes—out of tens of thousands of commercial chemicals—have ever been regulated.

Voluntary programs for self-monitoring and self-correction have proven inadequate, the American Academy of Pediatricians insisted, and chemical-management policy "needs to be rewritten." The new policy statement signaled physicians' growing frustration and confusion regarding numerous substances that have recently been revealed to be widespread in our homes, bodies and environment.

Many of these chemicals were originally touted as inert, harmless and safe. But new information reveals that many of these substances are far from benign.

Phthalates, for instance, are chemicals added to plastics to render them flexible. They were once believed to be completely inert, but it is now obvious that they leach readily from plastics and into foods, drinks, and the environment. It's more than a little troubling that phthalates have been documented in the bloodstreams of about 90% of Americans. Phthalates are present in everything from vinyl blood collection/storage bags, to children's toys, to women's cosmetics, hair sprays, nail polishes and perfumes. Alarmingly, a 2003 study concluded that phthalates are not only present in the bodies of a majority of Americans tested, but levels are highest among the most vulnerable group of all: women of childbearing age.

What's worse, these chemicals have been implicated in the obesity epidemic. Some pundits—and scientists—have taken to calling them "obesogens," meaning obesity-causing compounds. According to this emerging theory, the rising epidemic of obesity around the world may be traced to the widespread distribution throughout the environment (and our bodies) of chemicals that include BPA, phthalates, residues from nonstick cooking implements, and other chemicals.

This theory proposes that these hormone disruptors not only interfere with sexual maturation and reproduction, but they also affect hormonal signaling related to appetite regulation and "adipocyte biology." To put it more bluntly, these chemicals are suspected of interfering with the way our bodies metabolize and store fat, encouraging overeating and the runaway growth of fat cells in adults. Scientists have already discovered the specific biochemical pathways by which some of these chemicals promote obesity in animals, even when they are exposed to them while still developing in the womb.

Even more troubling is the interaction between these artificial chemicals and the endocrine receptors on cells throughout our bodies. These so-called endocrine disruptors mimic the action of human estrogens, with alarming implications for reproductive health and sexual maturation, among other concerns.

At a time when male infertility is on the rise around the world, and the incidence of once-uncommon conditions, such as autism spectrum disorder, is also skyrocketing, it seems unconscionable that we've allowed these potentially dangerous chemicals to run amok in our society. What's worse, these chemicals accumulate over time, possibly building to problematic levels.

A study conducted in Puerto Rico in 2000 examined the possible causes of an ongoing mystery. Why did a subset of Puerto Rican girls begin developing breasts at an extremely early age? The phenomenon had been documented nearly 20 years earlier.

The 2000 study examined blood levels of phthalates in 41 girls with early breast development, and an equal number of matched controls (girls with normal development). While it did not prove causation, the study found that the abnormally developing children had concentrations of a particular type of phthalate in their bloodstreams that was seven times higher than levels among control subjects. *Seven times* higher. And the average age of girls experiencing this early breast development? Two-and-a-half-years. *Two-and-a-half!*

Phthalate toxicity has also been linked to increased cardiovascular, liver and kidney disease. As the American Academy of Pediatrics statement illustrates, a big part of the problem we face as a nation is a glaring lack of knowledge. We don't always know where these substances are coming from, what harm they can do, how to avoid them, or how to eliminate them once ingested. Phthalates of several types are featured in common (and popular) air fresheners, for example.

BPA

Bisphenol A (BPA) is an organic compound used in the manufacture of certain widely-used types of plastic. Until recently, it was even found in plastic baby bottles. Studies have shown that these chemicals, which are added to plastics to make them pliable, are so ubiquitous in the modern environment that 95% of men, women and children have detectable levels in their bloodstreams.

"On the basis of results from recent studies using novel approaches to test for subtle effects, both the National Toxicology Program at the National Institutes of Health and FDA have some concern about the potential effects of BPA on the brain, behavior, and prostate gland in fetuses, infants, and young children," said the FDA in an update on BPA use, published in *Food Contact Application,* in January 2010.

BPA is among the highest-volume chemicals manufactured around the globe. We've known for decades that BPA is an endocrine disruptor. It tricks estrogen receptors into a state of inappropriate activation. Although we think of estrogens as female hormones, estrogen receptors are located throughout the bodies of both men and women, and play important roles in many normal functions.

Estrogen receptors are especially dense in nervous system and reproductive tissues, and animal studies suggest that their disturbance is likely to have an impact not only on individuals, but on individuals' offspring, even without direct exposure of the offspring to BPA. We've also known for decades that BPA leaches out of epoxy resins and polycarbonate plastics. This type of plastic is commonly used for bottled water, and in the lining of food cans, and studies have shown that BPA contamination of bottled water is likely to contribute significantly to an individual's burden of artificial endocrine disruptors.

More recently, scientists showed that ordinary house dust collected at locations throughout the Eastern United States contained measurable amounts of BPA. In fact, up to 95% of samples contained measurable amounts of BPA. The total contribution of BPA from indoor air exposure was estimated to be less than 1%, however, so this route is unlikely to be terribly significant. Even so, it's at least a little disturbing to discover that BPA is so common in the environment that even the air we breathe is now suspect. Concern over this shockingly widespread toxin has finally mounted to the extent that manufacturers are considering eliminating BPA from plastics used to store food or drink. Unfortunately, BPA-free alternatives presently available may contain chemical alternatives that are no better than BPA.

One, Bisphenol S (BPS), has already been shown to exhibit estrogenic effects, in some studies conducted abroad. The United States Environmental Protection Agency (EPA) is presently conducting tests on this and other alternatives. Another chemical in the bisphenol family, known as BPAF, is used in electronics and other applications. It is an even more powerful endocrine disruptor than BPA.

I find it disturbing that BPA has been detected on money. It's probably transferred there from receipts. Receipts are commonly printed on thermal paper these days, but this convenient technology is another source of BPA. Preliminary studies have shown that people who work with these receipts may absorb substantial amounts of BPA.

There's no clear solution to the widespread pollution of our bodies and our environment by these troubling endocrine disruptors, but there are a few steps one can take to reduce exposure. Skip the bottled water altogether, for example. Carry a metal reusable water bottle instead and refill it with filtered tap water. If you're a new parent, consider switching from baby bottles or bags to old-school glass baby bottles. Nearly as old as humankind, glass remains a toxin-free storage medium.

An article published in the journal *Alternative Medicine Review* cited data compiled by the Centers for Disease Control, which analyzed samples obtained nationwide as part of the National Health and Nutrition Examination Survey. Samples were obtained between 1999 and 2004, and included body fluids obtained from more than 7,000 individuals. In the majority of people tested, an alarming stew of toxic substances was detected. These included acrylamides, trihalomethanes, bisphenol A (BPA), phthalates, chlorinated pesticides, triclosan, organophosphate pesticides, pyrethroids, heavy metals, aromatic hydrocarbons, polybrominated diphenyl ethers, benzophenone from sunblock, perfluorocarbons from nonstick coatings, and numerous polychlorinated biphenyls and solvents.

As if all this evidence weren't enough, new findings were published in the September 2012 edition of the *Journal of the American Medical Association* (JAMA). Nearly three thousand participants, ranging in age from 6 to 19, were randomly selected for measurement of urinary BPA concentration. The results led researchers to conclude that BPA in urine was significantly associated with obesity.

So if you are trying to lose weight, but have been unable to do so, pay attention not only to what you eat, but to where and how your food has been stored. As I said before, BPA is found in foods and liquids that have been in contact with the chemical. Sources include everything from plastic bottles, to the lining of soup cans, to reusable plastic storage containers.

Heterocyclic amines (HCAs) are another example of potential carcinogens in our food. HCAs are formed when protein-rich foods, such as meats, are cooked at high, scorching temperatures. These compounds, most often present when charring is evident, have been linked to an increased risk of certain types of cancer.

Fortunately, presoaking meats in a marinade that features wine or some other plant-derived, high-antioxidant liquid, is an effective means of dramatically reducing the formation of these toxic chemicals. Of course, I might argue that eating less meat is also guaranteed to reduce this risk automatically.

Mercury and Lead

Mercury and lead are heavy metals that also pose a significant threat to health, and children are especially vulnerable. Exposure to these toxins has been linked to learning and behavior disorders, and may result in damage to multiple organ systems. Although humans have mined and made use of lead for millennia, scientists only recently concluded that there is no safe threshold for exposure to lead.

At the urging of public health experts, the United States government finally banned the widespread use of lead in paints and gasoline in the 1970s, but extensive damage had already been done. Lead from decaying paint in old buildings and contaminated soil is still a health threat decades later, especially among children from low-income families, as they are more likely to be exposed to this contaminant.

In fact, contaminated soil continues to contribute to a "shockingly high" incidence of lead poisoning in urban areas, according to a recent report by scientists at an American Midwestern university. Symptoms of lead poisoning in children may include hearing loss, delayed growth, clumsiness, and loss of newly acquired skills, such as speech.

Mercury is a metallic element that was once used widely in applications such as thermometers, blood pressure monitors and electric switches. Modern understanding of its extreme toxicity, however, has resulted in the banning of mercury for most such purposes. Nonprescription mercury-filled thermometers, for instance, were banned from sale beginning in 2003.

Acute exposure to mercury has been linked to a wide range of adverse health effects, including psychosis, hallucinations, tremors, delirium, insomnia, muscle spasms and even severe shyness. Higher blood levels have been linked to smoking and high consumption of fish and shellfish. Predator species of ocean fish, such as tilefish, swordfish, shark, king mackerel and albacore tuna, have all been shown to possess relatively high levels of methylmercury (the organic form of mercury), especially in muscle tissue, which is the edible portion of fish.

Mercury compounds are still used in some cosmetics, and some urban populations show surprisingly high blood levels of this poison. In New York City, for example, scientists with the city's department of health and mental hygiene conducted a study in 2004 to determine heavy metal levels among New York adults. Blood mercury levels were significantly higher than the national average, as were lead and cadmium levels. The heavy metal burden among some individuals was high enough to cause kidney damage. Another study found higher levels of mercury in the blood of people living in coastal areas of the United States, and the higher levels correlated with urbanites' higher consumption of problematic fish species.

Of course, one of the most notorious uses of mercury in modern history has been as a component of the chemical thimerosal. Although it was once commonly included as a preservative in vaccines, use of this controversial chemical has largely been discontinued.

Thimerosal was used successfully, and uneventfully, as a preservative for years, and it helped solve the potentially dangerous problem of bacterial contamination of vaccines. But in the late 1990s a group of scientists suggested that it might be associated with the development of autism among young children receiving the measles-mumps-rubella (MMR) vaccine. Even though a majority of scientists have rejected this association, there are reasons for concern.

Mercurochrome is another example of a once-common mercury-containing compound that has since been removed from the market. In the not-too-distant past, mercurochrome was a staple found in most Americans' medicine cabinets. Formerly used for the disinfection of minor wounds, mercurochrome has been effectively banned for sale in the United States since 1998.

Methylmercury

Methylmercury is an organic compound that is even more toxic than inorganic, elemental mercury, as it is more readily absorbed and incorporated into human tissues. It is strongly recommended that people limit their intake of predator species of ocean fish, including tilefish, swordfish, shark, king mackerel and albacore tuna. Pregnant or nursing mothers are advised to avoid eating these types of seafoods altogether. Contaminated ground water is another source of exposure, due primarily to the disposal of mercury-containing batteries in landfills.

Aluminum

Aluminum is an element; a light metal that, despite its relative abundance, serves no known function in biology. It has been linked to the degeneration of the brain, bone, and bone marrow (where most blood cells are produced). According to the latest research on the subject, aluminum is a neurotoxin (nerve poison) that interferes with more than 200 functions that are important for life. Indeed, this common metal is undergoing renewed scrutiny for its possible role in the development of Alzheimer's disease.

It may also be implicated in other neurodegenerative diseases, such as Parkinson's disease. Some of the sources of aluminum may surprise you. For example, some over-the-counter antacids still include aluminum compounds in their formulations. Likewise, many common antiperspirants and deodorants feature aluminum chlorohydrate. By applying these compounds to the skin daily, people unwittingly allow aluminum to get into the blood circulation.

This route of contamination is so significant that a recent study concluded that people with a long history of using aluminum-containing antiperspirants are significantly more likely to be diagnosed with Alzheimer's disease. Some research has also linked the use of aluminum-containing antiperspirants to an increased risk of breast cancer. Given that information, my advice is to avoid aluminum-based antiperspirant deodorants at all costs. Your body absorbs aluminum through the skin, allowing it to enter the bloodstream.

Get a free report on aluminum-free deodorants that I have personally tested by entering the key words "aluminum free deodorants" at CocoMarch.com.

Trans-Fats

Trans fats are still out there in numerous products, and should also be avoided at all costs. They are somewhat less of a concern now that market pressures have forced manufacturers to remove these artificial fats from most products. Although some trans fats occur naturally, the trans fats of concern to modern consumers are primarily artificial. These synthetic fat molecules have been cobbled together by food scientists working in laboratories to create shelf-stable artificial fats.

To me this is a classic example of how badly things tend to turn out when we allow technicians to dictate what goes into our food—and into our bodies—rather than relying on the wisdom of nature. Developed in the twentieth century to extend the shelf life of packaged foods, we now know that artificial trans fats are linked to a significantly increased risk of heart disease. Fortunately, these "designer" fats are nonexistent in my True Nutrition Plan.

Trans fats still appear in foods like prepackaged baked goods, so be on the lookout and avoid them whenever possible. Food manufacturers are required to list trans-fat content on product labels. But some products, such as in-house bakery goods, require only a list of ingredients.

Words to look for include "partially-hydrogenated" anything. "Partially-hydrogenated" is chemistry-speak for "artificial toxic fats." While both saturated fat and trans fats may raise "bad" LDL-cholesterol levels, trans fats have the additional disadvantage of simultaneously lowering "good" HDL-cholesterol levels. No wonder the National Academy of Sciences issued an advisory in 2002 stating that dietary trans fats represent a source of potential harm to consumers, while providing no known benefits.

Secrets to remember:

- Phthalates and BPA are likely to contribute significantly to an individual's burden of artificial endocrine disruptors, which may cause hormonal imbalances and weight gain.
- Avoid plastic water bottles and plastic containers. Do not eat canned soups; most cans have a lining that contains BPA.
- Read labels carefully. Avoid "partially hydrogenated" ingredients; these are trans fats. These man-made fats can increase your bad cholesterol levels, while lowering levels of good cholesterol.
- To get a free report on the most common food sources of hidden trans fats, go to my website. Enter the key words "trans fats" at CocoMarch.com.

CHAPTER 5

The Bitter Taste of Sugar

How sweet it is!
Jackie Gleason

W hile we're on the subject of substances that have negative effects on our lives, I should mention the prevalence of high fructose corn syrup (HFCS). HFCS was introduced in the mid-twentieth century as a byproduct of the corn industry.

It was touted as slightly sweeter and cheaper than table sugar (sucrose), which is primarily made from sugar cane. Food manufacturers embraced this new industrial sweetener. Americans were told that HFCS is perfectly safe. In fact, a recent advertising campaign promoted HFCS, claiming that sugar is sugar and your body doesn't know the difference, regardless of whether it's made from corn or sugar cane. I couldn't disagree more. As you will learn in this chapter, sugar may not be good for you, but sugar in the form of HFCS is even worse.

The corn industry still argues that their product is essentially the same as table sugar, but the science simply doesn't bear this out. Numerous studies (literally hundreds to date) have shown that the human body processes fructose differently than sucrose. It is clearly linked to the development of higher levels of uric acid in the bloodstream, for example. And elevated uric acid levels are directly linked to a higher incidence of painful gout, among other things.

Although it may conjure images of Medieval misery (Henry VIII was famously afflicted with gout, for example), gout is very much a modern disease. Like many lifestyle diseases, gout is on the rise in the United States. It is a condition in which uric acid forms needle-sharp crystals in the joints, resulting in crippling pain and inflammation. Treatment consists, not surprisingly, of dietary modifications, and inevitably, medications.

A recent study published in the prestigious *Journal of the American Medical Association* stated that drinking fructose-sweetened beverages was associated with an increased incidence of gout among the women participating in the long-term study. What's worse, high uric acid levels are now suspected of playing a role in the development of high blood pressure, kidney disease and cardiovascular disease.

Sweet Sorrow

A study published in 2008 followed the progress of thousands of men and women who showed no signs of the metabolic syndrome at initial enrollment, nearly three decades earlier. By 2003, subjects with the highest uric acid levels in their blood were significantly more likely to have the metabolic syndrome. Among female subjects, even a relatively modest spike in uric acid levels was associated with a two-fold higher risk of having the metabolic syndrome.

The study's authors concluded that higher levels of uric acid are a "strong and independent predictor" of metabolic syndrome in both men and women. This strikes me as highly significant, as the metabolic syndrome is linked to cardiovascular disease—still our *number one* killer.

HFCS is also "suspected" of playing a role in the rising incidence of type 2 diabetes, which, like obesity, is now epidemic in this country. I put "suspected" in quotation marks because the massively influential corn industry continues to exercise its considerable political powers of persuasion to strenuously refute this claim, and the medical establishment has been timid about accepting the obvious.

As a result, the popular press largely continues to perpetuate the myth that HFCS is of no special concern. But objective scientists working in independent laboratories at universities and other institutions around the world continue to publish data that adds up to only one logical conclusion: The rise in type 2 diabetes, obesity and the metabolic syndrome are almost certainly linked to the rise in consumption of HFCS—and the rise in sugar consumption in general—over the past few decades. Indeed, table sugar is not entirely benign by any means.

Fructose Versus Sucrose

Sucrose is composed of two simple sugars; glucose and fructose. So, while HFCS provides proportionally more fructose per serving, both are significant sources of fructose. As its name implies, fructose is a simple sugar primarily found in fruit. Studies have shown that fructose obtained from eating whole fruit poses no risk. This is probably because amounts are relatively small, or possibly because other natural substances in whole fruits—antioxidants and other phytonutrient compounds, for example—may counteract the effects of the fruit's fructose. In any event, the amount of fructose in the typical American diet is far greater than the amount supplied by a diet that incorporates reasonable amounts of fruits.

In fact, some scientists now believe that sugar is toxic. They point to changes in the number of cases of the metabolic syndrome, obesity and diabetes (sometimes called *diabesity*, because the two are so inextricably linked).

These changes have historically mirrored rising and falling consumption of sugar. This toxic effect evidently begins in the liver, where fructose is converted directly into fats, raising blood levels of compounds called triglycerides. High triglycerides are an independent risk factor for heart disease. They also cause a buildup of fat in the liver. This can result in a once-rare, but now increasingly common condition called non-alcoholic fatty liver disease. This constant pressure on liver function is also linked to the development of insulin resistance, another increasingly common condition. Insulin resistance is a condition in which the body's cells fail to respond appropriately to insulin.

Insulin is a hormone produced by specialized cells in the pancreas. It is released into the bloodstream in response to rising levels of glucose in the blood. Glucose is one of the primary sources of energy for cells. But if it is not rapidly shunted into the body's cells for processing, glucose can be damaging to blood vessels. Cell membranes are semi-permeable, meaning that many types of molecules may pass in and out, but not entirely freely. Insulin acts as a sort of shepherd for glucose, figuratively guiding glucose into the inner sanctum of the cell, where it is "burned" for energy production.

For some reason, when we eat too much sugar it encourages a cascade of abnormal and undesirable events. It begins with fat being deposited in the liver, then escalates to insulin resistance, and eventually leads to the development of type 2 diabetes. As cells increasingly fail to respond to insulin, glucose levels in the bloodstream continue to rise.

The pancreas attempts to compensate by cranking out still more insulin, but eventually it succumbs to "pancreatic exhaustion." In essence, insulin-producing cells "burn out" and the patient becomes an insulin-dependent diabetic. At this stage, a patient must rely on daily shots of insulin for survival.

To control rising and falling levels of glucose and insulin, these patients must monitor their blood sugar levels throughout the day, and attempt to adjust food intake and insulin doses accordingly. If blood sugar levels are allowed to rise to abnormally high levels for significant periods, long-term health suffers further.

Uncontrolled high blood sugar (hyperglycemia) damages blood vessels and fine nerves, eventually leading to conditions like peripheral neuropathy—a painful inflammation of the nerves that may manifest as tingling, numbness and outright pain—and increasingly poor circulation, especially in the extremities.

Some diabetics will eventually develop foot infections and recurrent foot ulcers. Some eventually lose their toes or feet. Other effects are no less unappealing, and include accelerated aging, declining sexual function and other problems.

Is Sugar Toxic?

As I mentioned, a new school of thought is gaining traction. It holds that sugar itself—no matter what form it takes—is toxic. Unlike more familiar acute toxins, like cyanide for instance, it doesn't kill quickly.

Rather, say proponents of the sugar-as-poison theory, it promotes the cascade of metabolic abnormalities described above, dramatically increasing risks for kidney disease, hypertension, type 2 diabetes, obesity, the metabolic syndrome, stroke, cardiovascular disease, and very likely, cancer. I believe this is undoubtedly true, but I also believe that HFCS is especially problematic.

In 2005, scientists based at the University of Toronto published an article in *Nutrition & Metabolism (London)*, in which they declared that excessive consumption of HFCS, primarily from sweetened soft drinks, represents a notable, but not well-appreciated change in dietary behavior.

Historically, per capita consumption of sugar, and fructose especially, was much lower than it is today. Furthermore, said the researchers, intake of high levels of fructose encourages increased production of fats and triglycerides by altering the manner in which the liver metabolizes glucose, the basic currency of energy for the body.

These metabolic disturbances may be at the root of increased insulin resistance, a condition that precedes full-blown type 2 diabetes. Accordingly, said the scientists, evidence from numerous studies "clearly suggests" that excess fructose consumption is a factor causing the rising epidemic of metabolic syndrome. The authors went on to suggest that more should be done to put the brakes on the food industry's use of high fructose corn syrup.

Other evidence strongly suggests that a high intake of HFCS contributes to kidney stone formation and the recent spike in cases of non-alcoholic fatty liver disease. As its name suggests, this is a condition in which the liver becomes dysfunctional and engorged with fat, much like the failing liver of a chronic alcoholic. But it happens despite the absence of alcoholism.

The drug of choice in this instance is evidently sugar—especially in the form of HFCS. The amount of HFCS in the U.S. food supply has risen from an estimated 16% of sweeteners in 1978 to 42% in 1998. Overall consumption of sugars of all types has also increased dramatically, largely driven by the popularity of sweetened soft drinks. Once regarded as a special treat, soft drinks are now consumed routinely by many Americans, and in portions that would probably have astounded previous generations.

The Puzzle

In my opinion sugar is a single piece of the puzzle that is the American diet. But it's a key piece. Sugar clearly plays a crucial role in the development of so-called western diseases. On May 26, 2009, Robert H. Lustig M.D. presented a lecture entitled "Sugar: The Bitter Truth". Lustig is a specialist in pediatric hormone disorders, and the leading expert on childhood obesity at the University of California. Watching the lecture online, I was surprised to hear Lustig refer to sugar as "evil." Evil is not the first word that comes to mind when thinking of sugar. No parent offers his or her child an ice cream cone, or a piece of candy, for instance, thinking I want to expose my child to evil.

Lustig makes it clear that when he uses the term sugar he is not just referring to what is commonly known as table sugar (sucrose), which is used in baking, or to sweeten coffee, for example. He's also referring to high-fructose corn syrup, which he calls "the most demonized food additive known to man."

The truth is that the number of obese and diabetic Americans has skyrocketed in the last few decades. Given that other chronic ailments have also increased, can excess sugar consumption be blamed?

Information is power, but misleading or incomplete information can create confusion. One example is the new wave of TV commercials encouraging you to buy soft drinks made with "real sugar." Consumers are catching up with researchers. Evidence shows that high-fructose corn syrup is bad for you. Soft drink manufacturers have responded by switching to sucrose. They've used this switch in new advertising that capitalizes on the "demonization" of HFCS. So confused buyers fall into the trap of thinking they are making better choices, since they're now avoiding high-fructose corn syrup.

But despite cynical marketing claims, the bottom line is that *no* added sugar at all is what's best for you. Lustig believes sucrose and HFCS are equally bad for you. In fact, he refers to them as "poisonous". Whether you consume sugar or high-fructose corn syrup your body has similar reactions, Lustig argues. To him, both are harmful. Unlike fruits, which are sweet but contain an array of naturally derived nutrients, refined sugar and HFCS don't have any nutrients, just calories from carbohydrates. None at all; no protein, vitamins, minerals, fiber or antioxidants.

Risky Calories

The more sugar we consume the fewer nutrient-rich foods we eat. For instance, if you have a breakfast that consists of coffee sweetened with sugar, and a donut or cookies, you are not eating a nutritious meal. You are missing an opportunity to eat something that provides your body nutrients, like a fruit smoothie, for example, and instead eating something that has an overall negative effect.

Why negative? When we eat foods that don't contain nutrients, they rob our body of existing substances such as calcium and other minerals, simply in order to pass through. Unlike natural plants, which provide most of what they need to be digested, sugar and HFCS create the opposite effect. And that is why they are called "empty calories".

Lustig takes the concept of "empty calories" a step further. Many scientists argue that a calorie is a calorie no matter where it comes from, and to some extent that is true. However, Lustig looks at the metabolic effects of calories when they are sourced from different foods. He says that metabolically the effect of a calorie can be greater than the calorie itself.

In fact, the sweet-flavored granular substance we call sugar is chemically composed of two basic monosaccharides. A monosaccharide (from the Greek *monos*: meaning single) is the basic unit of a carbohydrate. Sugar is made up of two different types of monosaccharides: 50% fructose and 50% glucose. On the other hand, HFCS is made up of 55% fructose. The remaining 45% is almost all glucose. I point this out because to understand the metabolic effect of different carbohydrates we need to know how our body metabolizes or digests them.

Fructose is primarily metabolized in the liver, while glucose is metabolized by virtually all cells in the body. If we consume foods high in fructose, such as sodas or candy, we're putting extra pressure on the liver. HFCS contains more fructose than granulated sugar (55% versus 50%). Therefore, the negative impact on the liver is even greater.

It is important to remember that the more granulated sugar we use and the more sodas loaded with HFCS we drink, the more glucose we consume, and this taxes the liver. But that's not all. An unnecessary amount of sugar can be defined as more than our body needs to burn for immediate energy usage. When the body has more sugar than it needs, much of the excess is transformed into fat by the liver.

This process, which requires excessive amounts of insulin to be continually pumped out, causes insulin resistance. Insulin resistance has been linked to obesity in many Americans. It may also play an important role in the development of heart disease and type 2 diabetes. Another risk factor is the metabolic syndrome. Having the metabolic syndrome is a major risk factor for heart disease and diabetes. It's no coincidence that diabetes and the metabolic syndrome are both ordinarily characterized by an expanding waistline. Being overweight means that you are very likely to suffer from the metabolic syndrome, which in turn makes you more likely to have a heart attack or to become diabetic.

Following my True Nutrition Plan will help you reduce your risk of developing the metabolic syndrome. It also helps you experience enhanced wellness and vibrant health. Over the years, I have met overweight patients who didn't seem to be experiencing a problem with diabetes yet. But I knew that in the absence of meaningful changes, many of these patients would succumb to the metabolic syndrome sooner or later. Many would have developed diabetes. It was just a matter of time, really, and depended on how much longer their pancreases could continue to crank out excessive amounts of insulin, before finally burning out.

Even if diabetes doesn't appear for many years, having persistently elevated insulin levels is nothing to aspire to. High blood sugar and insulin levels increase one's risk of heart disease due to higher triglyceride levels, high blood pressure, and, in most cases, low levels of "good" HDL-cholesterol and high levels of "bad" LDL-cholesterol.

Diabetes Hazard

So the question remains, what causes our cells to become resistant to insulin? A recent article published by Yale Scientific magazine, entitled "Research Links Sugar Consumption, Fat Production and Diabetes," noted that scientists at Yale School of Medicine, working with Dr. Varman Samuel, Assistant Professor of Endocrinology, recently uncovered a "feed-forward mechanism" linking dietary sugar to diabetes. This mechanism explains how excess sugar in the diet may lead to increased fat production in the liver and to the subsequent development of diabetes.

According to Samuel, depositing fat in the liver sets the stage for insulin resistance, by activating proteins that interfere with insulin signaling. And insulin resistance promotes type 2 diabetes. But what causes a fatty liver? Too much fructose. Fructose is readily converted into fat in the liver. Dr. Samuel refers to the newly described mechanism as a "feed-forward loop". "Feed-forward" is the opposite of *feedback*. Under normal conditions—meaning no excess fructose in the diet—our bodies do not deposit toxic amounts of fat in the liver.

High amounts of fructose in the bloodstream blinds the "feedback mechanism," prompting the liver to convert fructose to fat, which is then accumulated in the liver. Even small amounts of fat accumulating in the liver can perpetuate a chain reaction that causes increasingly more fat to be produced and stored in the liver.

Lustig and Samuel are no longer alone in raising the alarm about the dangers of sugar. In early 2012 the well know American television news magazine *60 Minutes* featured a segment focusing on Dr. Lustig's research. The report was hosted by Sanjay Gupta, M.D. Dr. Gupta is an American neurosurgeon and assistant professor of neurosurgery at Emory University School of Medicine, and associate chief on the neurosurgery service at Grady Memorial Hospital in Atlanta, Georgia. The piece was entitled "Is Sugar Toxic?"

In a later interview, Dr. Gupta cautioned that we should look at sugar consumption the same way we look at eating a greasy cheeseburger; it can cause heart disease and it's bad for you. Dr. Gupta's recommendation? Eat real foods, like fruits and vegetables. Minimize your visits to the inside aisles of the grocery store where all packaged food are found. Stick to the outer aisles of grocery stores, where fruits and vegetable are sold.

The solution? If sugar consumption is reduced or stopped, fat accumulation in the liver will also halt. Diabetes, most heart conditions, and obesity can disappear, and overall you will be healthier and live longer. How much sugar is too much sugar? Lustig advocates a balanced diet and recommends that women consume only 100 calories of added sugar per day; men no more than 150 calories. This is equivalent to 25 and 37.5 grams of sugar per day, respectively.

The Sugar table that follows can be used to calculate the amount of sugar found in one average serving of some popular foods. Keep in mind that most people do not consume only one serving. For example, the average home has 12-ounce cups in their kitchen cabinets. We tend to fill our cups accordingly, but the serving size provided by manufacturers is usually 8 fl oz. By using a larger serving size we may unwittingly consume greater amounts of sugar than intended. Keep portion sizes in mind when calculating sugar consumption.

Food	Serving Size	Grams of Sugar
Langers Grape Juice Plus 100% juice	8 fl ounces	36
V8 Fusion Vegetable Fruit 100% juice	8 fl ounces	26
Minute Maid Lemonade 12% Juice	8 fl ounces	29
Nesquick Fat Free Chocolate Milk	8 fl ounces	28
Kellogg's Smart Start Strong Heart	1 1/4 cup	17
Quaker Oatmeal Squares	1 cup	13
Quake Granola Oats & Honey & Raising	1 cup	26
Pop Tart, Chocolate Fudge	1 pastry	20
Little Debbie Swiss Rolls	2 cakes	27
Store Brand Chocolate Chip Muffins	1 muffin	32
Hostess Ho Hos	3 cakes	42
Average Frozen Yogurt	1 cup	37

With even a cursory glance at this table, it's obvious how easy is to consume an excessive amount of sugar. An 8-fl oz cup of any juice contains more than 30 grams of sugar. If all the added sugar we consumed in one day came from just one 8-ounce cup of juice, we would already have exceeded Dr. Lustig's recommendation of 100 sugar calories per day, or less, for women, and would have nearly reached the 150 calorie limit for men.

I highly discourage drinking fruit juices. If you insist on serving fruit juice to your children, mix 2 fl ounces of juice with 10 fl oz of water.

Children will get used to that and if you train them from an early age, you can reduce sugar intake to 9 grams or less. This is important, because besides obvious sugars, from sources that are evident, we also need to account for hidden sources of sugar. These include foods such as bread, sauces, salad dressings, ketchup and many others.

This might seem overly restrictive if you are used to consuming sugar freely, without paying much attention to amounts. But the benefit is clear. Stop eating granulated sugar and HFCS, and the threat of fatty liver disease goes away, and with it the specter of insulin resistance and may of the other conditions I have already discussed.

 ## Secrets to remember:

- Replace sugar ordinarily added to coffee or beverages with a natural non-sugar choice like Truvia® or stevia.
- Replace sodas with filtered water. Add natural flavors if you like. You can find liquid natural and organic flavorings near the spices in your grocery.
- If you dislike the taste of water drink a couple of sips of juice after you are done.
- Dilute juice with filtered water: 2 fl oz of juice with 10 fl oz of filtered water. Add a couple drops of stevia if it is not sweet enough.
- Read labels.

To get a free report on ways to reduce your sugar consumption, visit my website and download my free report. Enter the key words "less sugar" at CocoMarch.com.

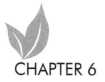

CHAPTER 6

Creating a Safe Home

*Here's kind of my motto—if you're not happy
at home, you're not happy anywhere else.*
Angie Harmon

Any old place I can hang my hat is home sweet home to me.
William Jerome

Home is where we feel safe, protected and comfortable. Even after a long awaited vacation, most of us are delighted to get back home. Home is more than a place to dwell, it is a refuge. But security at home requires more than just a stout front door with a sturdy lock. A solid roof overhead may protect us from torrential rains, but what about less obvious threats? Could it be that unseen dangers lurk behind the comforting facades of our modern homes?

The simple answer is yes. In the past few decades scientists have accumulated evidence that many of the objects, products and furnishings we've taken for granted may be far less benign than we once believed. Many of these products were touted as revolutionary

45

improvements. As it turns out, some of that convenience comes at a cost. And the cost may be greater than you think.

Non-stick Cookware

Non-stick cookware is a prime example. It features a synthetic thermoplastic polymer, polytetrafluoroethylene (best known as Teflon®), which renders cookware less prone to sticking, and therefore easier to clean. While the chemical industry claims that non-stick cookware is perfectly safe, at high temperatures polytetrafluoroethylene-based coatings may release fluorocarbon gases (collectively called perfluorochemicals). When inhaled, these gases have been linked to flu-like symptoms in humans, and they've been known to kill birds outright. Despite these findings, some manufacturers even coat microwave popcorn bags with these compounds. Alarmingly, researchers with the New York Department of Health showed in 2007 that some commercially available microwave popcorn bags release problematic perfluorochemicals during normal use.

Some of these chemicals are believed to be endocrine disruptors, and some have been identified as likely human carcinogens by the United States Environmental Protection Agency's Science Advisory Board. They've also been shown to damage animals' livers and kidneys, and to interfere with reproduction and immunity. In one study, Swedish researchers found that concentrations of perfluorochemical pollutants were higher in people who reported eating the most fast food, evidently due to manufacturers' use of the compounds in food packaging. Grease-resistant paper, for example, may contribute to exposure.

It's unclear what negative effects these chemicals may have on human health. Nevertheless, it's chilling to think that these synthetic compounds are accumulating in the blood and tissues of humans and animals all over the world. Environmental contamination is so widespread, these chemicals have even been detected in remote polar regions.

According to the EPA, low doses of these chemicals have been found circulating in the bloodstreams of most Americans. A 2006 study conducted in New York concluded that perfluorochemical pollution was widespread in a sampling of bodies of water throughout the state. The compounds were common in the tissues of fish and fowl.

Avoiding non-stick cookware may be insufficient to reduce one's exposure, given that these chemicals are widespread in the environment. Nevertheless, I recommend avoiding the use of non-stick cookware. It may seem daunting at first to ban non-stick cookware from your kitchen, but I believe it's worthwhile. To reduce your daily exposure to these questionable chemicals you must embrace cooking technology that our grandmothers would recognize: iron and stainless steel cookware.

If you are not accustomed to cooking with stainless steel, there may be a bit of a learning curve as you master new techniques (or old ones, depending on your perspective) to help prevent sticking and to keep cookware clean and shiny. One trick is to replace cooking oils with vegetable, chicken or beef stock. Doing so will not only reduce the total calories you consume (remember that each tablespoon of fat represents about 120 calories). This will also help prevent foods from sticking to the bottom of the pan.

Another trick is to rinse your pans immediately after cooking. Add water with a bit of non-foaming soap and put the pan *back on the stove*. Let it heat up while you enjoy dinner. By the time you're done eating, simply pour the hot water into the sink. With the scrubby side of a sponge, wash out any food still adhering to the pan. You will be amazed by how little work you'll have to do to keep pans clean. For stubborn food residue you can sprinkle a bit of baking powder onto the pan, spray some white vinegar, and rub, using a more abrasive sponge.

Visit my website and download my free manual on how to cook on stainless steel. Enter the key words "stainless steel" at CocoMarch.com.

Hand Soap

Antibacterial chemicals, such as triclocarban, are found in many soaps and house cleaners. These chemicals are problematic in that they are persistent in the environment and they may contribute to our bodies' load of foreign chemicals. Studies show that these compounds do more harm than good, as they encourage microbes to develop resistance and become still more virulent. By using these common products, people may inadvertently encourage the very thing they had hoped to avoid: the spread of virulent pathogens capable of causing illness.

Other studies have consistently shown that washing hands with non-antibacterial soap (good, old-fashioned soap) is just as effective at reducing the spread of respiratory and gastrointestinal illnesses as antibacterial hand soap. Without the unnecessary chemicals.

That's because hand washing has always worked to reduce the spread of illness through the simple, mechanical action of physically removing germs from the skin surface and washing them away. In fact a meta-analysis conducted in 2008 looked at data from numerous clinical trials, and concluded that the most effective approach to thwarting the spread of certain communicable illnesses is education about the importance of hand washing with ordinary soap.

I recommend using organic soaps that are made from natural oils. Castile soap is said to be named for the region of "Castilla" in Spain, and it's my favorite. Originally, Castile Soap was made from olive oil, but now the term castile soap refers to soaps made with fat purely of vegetable origin. If it is organic, all the fats are of organic origin, including any essential oils added to provide scent. My favorite brand is Dr. Bronner's Magic Pure Castile Soap, Eucalyptus. I like the refreshing feeling I get after using it to shower. It also comes in a number of other natural essences, such as rose, lemon, peppermint, and so on.

Shampoo and Conditioner

An article published in the *American Journal of Epidemiology* by Johns Hopkins University School of Hygiene and Public Health alerted consumers about the chemical dangers lurking in products that we apply to our hair. Researchers noted that some of the chemicals used in various hair treatments may be absorbed through the skin of women and their infants. Their findings suggested that toxic chemicals can be absorbed through the scalp in amounts sufficient to trigger "...a variety of adverse health effects."

Although much more research is required to determine the full extent of any negative effects these chemicals may have, I believe in the motto "better safe than sorry." Which is why I suggest you use only botanical shampoos and conditioners. I realize that initially they may not seem to work as well as synthetic chemical-based products, but I have done the homework for you. I recommend Trader Joe's Tea Tree Tingle Shampoo with Peppermint, Tea Tree and Eucalyptus Botanicals. I also highly recommend Tea Tree Tingle conditioner. I recommend it because I like the ingredients; it smells natural and it's quite affordable. In fact, it's an excellent value. Some of the natural oils and botanicals in this product include tea tree, peppermint, eucalyptus, rosemary, nettle, thyme, birch leaf, chamomile, clary, lavender, coltsfoot leaf and yarrow oil.

Visit my website and download my free report on the best natural soaps and shampoos I have found. Enter the key words "clean body" at CocoMarch.com.

Sunscreen

We have been indoctrinated to believe that exposure to the sun is dangerous. We've been taught that sunscreens are essential to protect our children from burns, which might lead to skin cancer in the future. This makes sense, but there are two potential problems with this sun-avoidance obsession. One: We all need some minimal, unimpeded sun exposure to produce crucially important vitamin D. And two: Most presently available sunscreens contain potentially harmful chemicals.

Most sunscreens contain chemicals, such as oxybenzone. This common UV filter chemical is an endocrine disruptor that may seep into children's bloodstreams, where it can interact with estrogen receptors throughout the brain and body. No one knows for sure what effect this might have on development and maturation. Mineral-based UV filters, such as zinc oxide or titanium dioxide are considered safer choices, as they do not penetrate the skin.

When purchasing a sunscreen for you and your family, read labels carefully and pay close attention to each ingredient, making sure it doesn't contain parabens (chemical preservatives), petrochemicals, phthalates, sulfates, propylene glycol, animal ingredients, synthetic fragrances, or dyes.

These days you can find many plant and mineral-based sunscreens at your local grocery and drug store in the natural section. If not, check the local health food store. Staff tend to be knowledgeable and friendly, and they can help you make good choices. I do not presently have a preferred sunscreen. In fact, most of the time, I don't use any. I try to limit my sun exposure to the later hours of the day, when the sun is less intense and doesn't burn as much.

If you have a favorite all-natural choice for sunscreen send me a message via my website, at CocoMarch.com. I will research it and add it to my list of recommendations if it meets my criteria for safety and effectiveness.

Paint

Other toxins of concern are found nearly everywhere. As I noted earlier, volatile organic compounds (VOCs) are one class. Emitted by paints and plastics, they have been linked to adverse health effects. Fortunately, you can now find many paints that are low-VOC or even VOC-free. When painting my house, I used Sherwin-Williams paints. I was impressed by the quality of their "Green Sure" line, which is free of VOCs. I found it remarkable to be able to enter a just-painted room and not smell the familiar paint odors that signal the presence of toxic VOCs.

Carpeting

A recent report by the British Society for Allergy & Clinical Immunology noted that it is likely that increased exposure to synthetic and pollutant chemicals contributes substantially to increases in allergic disease. Chemicals like organotins, permethrin, triclosan, formaldehyde, polybrominated diphenyl ether, flame retardants and phthalates are used in the manufacture of synthetic carpeting. I recommend using wool carpeting, or carpets made from corn byproducts. The latter are becoming increasingly popular and will reduce your exposure to these harmful chemicals.

Visit my website to download a free report on tips to reduce VOC levels at home. Enter the key words "safe remodel" at CocoMarch.com.

Laundry Detergent

Laundry detergents contain chemicals such as chlorine and phosphates. Phosphates are known water pollutants containing the element phosphorus. Phosphates have caused considerable environmental damage in the last few decades. As phosphate compounds leach into lakes and streams, these chemicals encourage the runaway growth of algae. This, in turn, depletes oxygen levels in the water. This can lead to oxygen starvation among the organisms that normally live in the water. Thus, phosphates from detergent contribute to the death of fish and plants, and can throw entire ecological systems out of balance.

Organic or naturally derived laundry detergent does not contain harsh chemicals, dyes and perfumes that may be dangerous to our health, or to the health of the environment. Consider replacing your conventional laundry detergent with organic laundry soap. If you can't find it in your local grocery or health food store, look for it online, or purchase the simple ingredients and make your own. You'll be surprised that the cost is not much higher, but the benefits to your heath are considerable. In fact, many people make their own laundry soap from simple ingredients such as washing soda, borax and pure hand soap, for less money than they would spend on commercially available laundry detergents.

Dry Cleaning

Even the way we dry clean our clothes may affect our exposure to potentially harmful toxins. Dry cleaning, for instance, uses organic solvents. One of the most common is tetrachloroethylene, commonly called "perc." It is classified as a hazardous material by the EPA.

Alternatives are arguably less problematic, but still emit volatile organic compounds (VOCs), which contribute to air pollution. A new process that uses liquid carbon dioxide is considerably more environmentally friendly, but it costs at least twice as much as conventional dry cleaning and it's not always as effective as older methods.

To reduce your exposure to these organic compounds, it's helpful to remove plastic bags from cleaned clothes before you bring the clothes into the home. Don't take them to your closet and hang them up right away, otherwise these invisible, practically odorless substances will become airborne in your home as soon as you remove the plastic.

Allow clothes to air out—outdoors if possible—or if it's too cold, just do it in the garage. Leave them for a day or two before taking them indoors. By doing this you will reduce your exposure to dry cleaning VOCs by more than 90%.

Cigarette Smoke

For some Americans cigarette smoke still represents a clear and present danger to the health not only of the smoker, but of his or her loved ones as well. Children raised in homes with at least one smoker are at increased risk of asthma, ear infections, and other respiratory ailments, for example. And new information indicates that there is simply no safe level of exposure to secondhand smoke. None. Period. This has been determined using gene assays on tissue samples taken from people with varying degrees of smoke exposure.

Even people with barely detectable exposure to cigarette smoke showed signs of changes in the genes of cells lining the airways. These changes are believed to precede the development of diseases such as chronic obstructive pulmonary disease (COPD) and lung cancer. So, viewed another way, smoking cessation represents a golden opportunity to improve the health of an entire household.

Like obesity, smoking is an independent risk factor for numerous degenerative diseases. It increases oxidative stress, inflammation, and the risk of developing cardiovascular disease. Smoking is also linked to an increased risk of developing various types of cancer. Lung cancer is the most obvious of these, but smoking has been linked to an increased risk of numerous other types of cancer as well.

According to the results of a study published by Japanese researchers, obese men and women who smoke *and* have symptoms of diabetes are at increased risk of developing atherosclerosis, regardless of age. Subjects who smoked and had abnormally high levels of insulin showed signs of increased plaque buildup within the vessel walls of a major artery. This measurement is considered an accurate indicator of both present and future atherosclerosis. Smoking is especially risky for diabetic patients, therefore, because smokers develop advanced atherosclerosis sooner than people with standard risk factors alone.

 ## Secrets to remember:

- Never cook with non-stick cookware.
- Avoid antibacterial soaps.
- Avoid synthetic personal and household cleaners.

Visit my website to get a free report on tips for safe household cleaning. Enter the key words "natural cleaners" at CocoMarch.com.

PART II

Personal Application

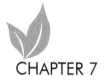

CHAPTER 7

You Are
What You Eat

We need to take responsibility for our bodies, and food is the first step.
Cocó March

You don't have to cook fancy or complicated masterpieces,
just good food from fresh ingredients.
Julia Child

During the years I practiced medicine in the United States, patients with a wide variety of ailments came to me for help. My patients' problems ranged from the mundane to life-threatening. Before long, I said this before but I will repeat it, in most cases patients' problems, such as obesity, diabetes, heart disease and even cancer, could be traced back to the lifestyle habits of the past decade or so of a given patient's life.

Invariably, these patients had eaten poorly, shirked exercise and allowed their body weight to climb well past the point of ideal. It was

57

no wonder they ended up with serious illnesses. My formal training and personal life experience had shown me that diet and health are intimately linked.

While most Americans are at least intellectually aware that certain foods and eating habits are not "good for them," I got the impression that Americans still tend to disregard the seriousness of the relationship between what we put in our bodies and how our bodies react. It seems to me that few people truly grasp the power of food to affect overall health until they are dangerously sick.

As bad as that effect can be when diet is poor—witness the obesity epidemic— food's effect on health can be equally positive, given the right food choices enjoyed in appropriate amounts. Thus, much of my work with these patients involved educating—or reeducating them, in some cases—about diet. I taught them to rethink their approach to food, and to re-imagine food's role in their lives.

More than two thousand years ago, the ancient Greek physician who would become known as the "father of Western medicine," wrote these timeless words of wisdom: "Let food be thy medicine; let medicine be thy food."

It turns out that Hippocrates knew so many centuries ago what many of us have forgotten: Food is more than mere sustenance; it provides the means to sustain not just life, but wellness. Here was a European with a plan! His idea was to recognize the power of food to engender wellness and encourage healing.

You may wonder, if our diets have changed so drastically for the worse in the past three or four generations, why have average lifespans increased so dramatically in that time? The answer is simple: they haven't. Yes, the average male or female baby born today is estimated to live until about 80 years of age. And the average male or female born in 1900 had a life expectancy of about 50. But these numbers are misleading.

In 1900, infant mortality was exceptionally high. Today it is low. A majority of people died of infectious or communicable diseases in 1900. Today chronic diseases are much more likely to be the cause of death. If you account for the changes in infant mortality rates between 1900 and 2000, you will see that the change in "healthspan," or the time a person lives in a state of good health, is probably decreasing, rather than increasing.

In some countries—notably Greece, where adherence to the Mediterranean diet was exceptionally high before World War II— mortality rates among some groups are actually increasing. Men in these countries, for instance, have experienced a 20% to 40% increase in deaths from cardiovascular disease. This is likely due to "modernization" of the diet there, meaning more exposure to prepared and fast foods, and less adherence to a traditional, remarkably healthful Mediterranean diet. The diet relies heavily on whole grains, vegetables, fruits, nuts, fresh herbs, olives, fish and some dairy. Meat is often used for little more than flavoring. In the early twentieth century, heart disease was virtually unheard of in most Mediterranean countries. That is no longer true.

Changes in the dietary habits of the region's populations, in the wake of World War II, have been identified as a likely source of this disturbing trend. Similarly, Japanese citizens enjoy remarkably good health, with lower rates of cancer, heart disease, hypertension and diabetes, than in the West.

But studies have repeatedly shown that when Asians move to the United States and adopt our diet and lifestyle, these health advantages begin to disappear very quickly. This is surely no coincidence. The traditional diet of the Japanese people, as typified by Okinawa islanders, consists primarily of seaweed (a highly nutritious vegetable), vegetables, seafood and rice. Indeed, residents of Okinawa who still eat as their ancestors have for centuries are among the longest-lived people on the planet.

Paradoxically, improvements in nutrition are believed to have played a role in some of the gains in lifespan that have been documented in Western countries throughout the twentieth century. Food is cheaper, and more widely available, and preservation methods are less likely to rely on salt than in 1900. So more people have better, more continuous access to nutritious food than in 1900. There is also better understanding about specific nutritional deficiencies related to particular nutrients. For example, illnesses directly linked to too little dietary niacin, or vitamin B3 (pellagra), thiamine, or vitamin B1, (beriberi), and insufficient vitamin D (rickets), are no longer rampant.

But there has also been a trend away from eating whole foods, fresh foods, and locally grown foods. Arguably, the increased affordability and availability of food has saved many from malnutrition and outright starvation. But it has also encouraged excess calorie consumption and surely plays a role in the unprecedented epidemic of overweight and obesity in the developed world.

Ironically, while we are better fed and less likely to suffer food deprivation than any previous generation in history, many of us are nevertheless suffering from malnutrition. After all, good nutrition depends on far more than access to calories. It also requires balance.

If an individual eats little more than hamburgers and fries every day, washed down with sugary sodas, he will certainly get plenty of calories. Probably too many. But will he balance those calories with an adequate intake of vitamins, minerals, trace elements, fiber and antioxidants? Certainly not.

And that's a prescription for any number of nutrition related ailments. Hence my skepticism that modern Americans' lifespans are truly increasing. A study conducted by United States-based researchers examined a wide range of data and tentatively concluded that the age-specific health status of the American population remains relatively unchanged.

Meat

In past centuries in most Mediterranean countries, meat animals—primarily goats, sheep and poultry—were free-range grazers. Unlike American supermarket offerings, these animals were typically not fattened on corn. This is notable, because corn is a source of pro-inflammatory omega-6-fatty acids, while grass and forage are rich sources of naturally anti-inflammatory omega-3 fatty acids.

Food animals that are allowed the freedom to graze as nature intended are naturally lower in fat. They also provide a higher proportion of healthful fats than meat from grain-fed, factory-farmed animals, which is typically what is sold to American consumers. Perhaps more disturbing is the fact that feedlot beef must be treated with antibiotics. This is because cattle are not adapted to eating solely grains. They evolved to derive nutrition from grasses.

Totally indigestible to most mammals, grasses are fermented in a special digestive chamber, where beneficial bacteria work to release the plants' nutrients. Nontypical foods, such as corn, overwhelm this system and potentially cause illnesses. Resulting diet-related maladies are prevented and/or treated with massive doses of antibiotics.

All of this is done to fatten the animals to an unnatural degree before slaughter. As a result of these practices, modern factory-farmed beef is not only higher in saturated fat and lower in beneficial omega-3 fatty acids than grass-fed beef, it also carries a steep price for long-term public health. New strains of dangerous *e. coli* and salmonella bacteria, capable of infecting and harming humans, have been linked to this unnatural, but exceptionally common practice of forcing unnatural foods on cattle. Because the classic Mediterranean diet features scant beef, it provides remarkably little saturated, artery-clogging fat, let alone toxic trans-fats.

Meat, Dairy and Your Health

This book is not about veganism or how to become a vegan. Rather, it is intended to help you achieve better health. But achieving better health requires changes. Some of these changes include replacing less healthy foods with more healthful ones. If what you are accustomed to doing has not yielded excellent health, there's still time to make positive changes that will help you look and feel better.

As you will learn, my plan accepts most natural foods. Organic meat, whether it's poultry or beef, is certainly natural. But I also want to share with you what science has revealed about reducing one's intake of meat and dairy products. I encourage the consumption of a variety of healthful foods, not just animal proteins, as some diet plans that have come in and out of fashion in the past few decades have done. I find those to be unrealistic and unhealthy for long term use.

It could be argued that Leonardo da Vinci was one of the world's first proponents of a diet free of meat. Da Vinci was a genius for the ages. His inventiveness and imagination gave flight to an astounding number of brilliant ideas. Here was a European man, born in humble circumstances in Tuscany, who retired to a private mansion in France, the honored guest of King Francois I. Da Vinci died peacefully at his lovely manor, le Clos Lucé, in Amboise, in 1519. He was 67.

In the mid-fifteenth century, when da Vinci was born, life expectancy for a male child was less than half the age he ultimately attained. I think the reason the master artist/inventor/scientist beat the odds had a lot to do with his diet. Da Vinci was a vegetarian. Growing up in relatively humble circumstances in Tuscany, he was undoubtedly exposed to the traditional Mediterranean diet, with its heavy emphasis on local fruits, vegetables and grains.

As his wealth increased, he might well have eaten far more meat. In Medieval society, especially in northern territories, those who could afford it commonly ate a great deal of meat. More affordable vegetables were considered peasant food among some societies at the time. But da Vinci declined to eat meat. Indeed, he abhorred the idea of eating animal flesh.

"Truly man is the king of beasts," Da Vinci wrote, "for his brutality exceeds theirs. We live by the death of others: we are burial places! I have from an early age abjured the use of meat, and the time will come when men such as I will look on the murder of animals as they now look on the murder of men."

Clearly, da Vinci was a committed vegetarian who felt a strong moral imperative to reject meat for sustenance. I'm not saying you have to be a strict vegetarian to improve your health. Nor do I appeal to you to make the switch towards a more vegetarian lifestyle on moral grounds. My reasons are somewhat less altruistic: I encourage you to broaden your consumption of fruit and vegetables, not necessarily to become a vegan but because it's better for *you*.

I was raised as an ovo-lacto-vegetarian, meaning we were vegetarians who also ate occasional eggs and low-fat dairy products. I think it's fascinating that da Vinci had this little-noticed passion for pure vegetarianism. His reasons were philosophical, but perhaps he suspected it would help him live longer, too. If so, this is just another example of his remarkable ahead-of-his-time thinking.

Da Vinci's vegetarianism was rooted in ideology, but scientists researching the effects of meat and dairy consumption on the human body in the past few decades have reached similar conclusions based on observation and study. For example, studies conducted by T. Colin Campbell, Ph.D. and Caldwell B. Esselstyn, Jr., M.D., show that vegetarianism may simply be healthier. Campbell and Esselstyn point out in their book, and documentary film, *Forks Over Knives*, that many types of cancer, arteriosclerosis and heart disease are minimal or nonexistent in countries that have never adopted a Western-style diet.

This remarkable book and film, which you can stream online, shines light on an undeniable conclusion: Increased consumption of animal and dairy products is closely related to an increased risk of heart disease. In the film, Dr. Esselstyn notes that during the occupation of Norway by the Germans during World War II, the invaders confiscated all the livestock and farm animals to provide supplies for their own troops. This forced the Norwegians to eat a plant-based diet.

The statistics presented by Dr. Esselstyn in the documentary are irrefutable. Despite the deprivations forced on the people, heart attack and stroke in Norway plummeted. As soon as things returned to normal, however—and meat, dairy products and sugar were reintroduced to the populace—strokes and heart attacks returned to pre-war levels.

In the meantime, in the Philippines, T. Colin Campbell, PhD was investigating the connection between animal and dairy consumption and our most deadly diseases. John McDougall, MD, who in the mid-1970s practiced medicine on a sugar plantation in Hawaii, also came to the same conclusion as Esselstyn.

Dr. McDougall noticed the health of the people on the sugar plantation differed depending on how long they had lived in Hawaii. He saw that people who had been raised in Japan, the Philippines, Korea and China, were invariably slim. These first-generation Asians also enjoyed a remarkable freedom from heart disease, prostate cancer, colon cancer, breast cancer, rheumatoid arthritis and multiple sclerosis. Overweight and obesity were virtually absent, too. People in their eighties and nineties were not invalids. On the contrary, they enjoyed full mobility and functionality. Their children were another story, though. The longer they lived in the West, the fatter and sicker they became. By the third generation kids were "as fat and sick as anyone I had seen," says McDougall.

As he expresses in the film, it became clear to McDougall that the striking difference between first generation Asians and their descendants was diet. First generation Asians were raised on a typical diet of rice and vegetables in their native land. But their children had adopted the dietary pattern of their new homeland. They abandoned rice and vegetables, substituting animal foods and dairy products. McDougall says the results were clear, as these kids became just as sick and overweight as everyone else.

Even though at the time of their discoveries Campbell, Esselstyn, and McDougall didn't know of each other's research, they ultimately reached a similar, revolutionary conclusion: Eating a simple, whole foods, plant-based diet can eliminate many of our most crippling conditions and diseases. Their consensus conclusion was profound. To put it succinctly: The foods we eat cause most diseases.

Veganism is generally recognized for its ability to reduce the risks of developing everything from obesity and heart disease, to cancer and kidney disease. A well planned vegan diet is associated with protection from many infirmities, but there are potential pitfalls if one is not careful.

The danger of veganism is that some people who become vegan do not necessary become healthy. Let me explain. The definition of veganism is: "The practice of abstaining from the use of animal products". The question is, why are some vegans not "healthy?"

Some who join the ranks of veganism do it not by switching to a plant-based diet, but by simply replacing their animal-based junk food consumption with non-animal-based junk foods. I don't want to generalize, but I have to point out that to not eat meat, or to minimize the amount of meat one eats, is not the only step necessary in order to acquire good health.

I have met many "vegetarian junkies" who live on pasta, bread, baked goods, and ready-made microwavable meals. Such vegans are not doing themselves much good. These are the vegans who are overweight and as sick as any meat eater. But why? Their diets are not rich in plants. They consume an abundance of refined carbohydrates, which supply very few vitamins, minerals and antioxidants, as well as little or no protein.

But even well-intentioned plant-based vegans must take care to get adequate amounts of certain nutrients that are crucial for complete nutrition, such as vitamin B_{12}, iron, calcium, iodine, vitamin D, complete protein and omega-3 fatty acids. For example, omega-3 fatty acids—especially docosahexaenoic acid (DHA) and eicosapentaenoic acid (EPA)—are found in abundance in cold-water fatty fish, such as tuna and wild salmon.

Plants only supply a third form, alpha-linolenic acid (ALA). And plant sources of ALA are relatively few at that. ALA can be obtained from foods such as flaxseed or walnuts (or the new fad, chia seeds), and then ALA is converted in the body to the essential nutrients DHA and EPA. Due to this conversion, which is fairly inefficient, veganism can have its challenges. But a well planned vegan diet, rich in grains, legumes, fruits and vegetables, supplies a plentitude of those nutrients.

According to research published in the *Journal of Nutrition*, increased red meat consumption has been associated with a greater risk of developing the metabolic syndrome, and with higher levels of C-reactive protein, a blood marker of chronic inflammation.

The metabolic syndrome is a cluster of conditions that predict cardiovascular disease risk. These conditions include hypertension, high blood sugar and/or insulin resistance, high blood lipid levels, elevated C-reactive protein levels and visceral obesity.

Researchers surveyed nearly 500 women, ranging in age from 40 to 60, to determine the relationship between their red meat consumption and the risk of developing the metabolic syndrome. Subjects' blood lipids, blood pressure, blood glucose and C-reactive protein levels were measured. The subjects were assigned to one of five groups, based on their reported red meat intakes. Subjects reporting the highest intake of red meat were significantly more likely to have the metabolic syndrome than subjects in the lowest intake category. Meat eaters also had higher levels of C-reactive protein, indicating they had relatively increased inflammation.

As we have seen, excess sugar consumption—which according to Dr. Lustig is equivalent to as little as 25 grams of sugar a day for a female—is the culprit behind diabetes, the metabolic syndrome and much heart disease. Research supports the notion that the effects of a high intake of red meat have similar results. These are strong indicators that reducing one's sugar and meat consumption may be more beneficial than we can imagine.

Give Up All Meat?

When reading all this information you may think that you have to give up all meat. But if this is not appealing to you, don't feel discouraged. You don't have to be vegan in order to be healthier. Although veganism can be great, not everyone is ready to make such a switch. To become a healthier you, you simply must do better than you've been doing so far. And you can do that by making just a few changes.

Start by only eating certified organic or free range meats from animals that have been raised on a healthy grass diet, and have not been treated with hormones or antibiotics. Animals that are allowed to forage freely have fewer diseases and get sick less often. You don't necessarily have to give up red meat, but try consuming it less frequently. The thought of doing so may be overwhelming, but it is doable.

Tapering

If you are accustomed to eating meat and potatoes daily, as many Americans are, asking you to only eat beef occasionally may seem like a challenging task. The good news is that you don't have to completely cut it out of your life; you just have to be moderate in how much you consume and reduce your intake slowly. Start by tapering off slowly. Begin by cutting your portions in half. If you would normally eat a large steak, try eating a smaller one, or share a bigger one with someone else.

You should get used to eating smaller portions of red meat over time. It can take as many as three to six months to become accustomed to reducing your portion sizes and to be satisfied with it. Once you are used to eating half as much red meat as you once did, reduce how often you eat it. If you ate red meat three to five times per week, cut the frequency in half for a couple of months, then cut it in half again, until you eating meat just once a week. Maintain your weekly red meat meal for at least six months.

Ideally, after one year you will be ready to eat meat only once every ten days or so. In the meantime, you will be adding new foods to your diet. As you increase the variety of foods you eat, you'll find that you're less likely to miss eating meat and potatoes at virtually every meal.

Secrets to remember:

- Veganism is not always healthy. If you chose to be a vegan, learn how to be a healthy one.
- Occasional red meat is permissible. If you are currently eating too much, taper down your intake over a period of months.
- Make sure to buy only Certified Organic meats.

For a list on a variety of meals that are not only rich and healthy but that are also tasty and simple to prepare. Visit my website and download my free recipes. Enter the key words "quick meals" CocoMarch.com.

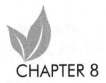

CHAPTER 8

Inactivity is Lethal!

If you don't take care of your body, where will you live?
Anonymous

Walking is the best possible exercise. Habituate yourself to walk very far.
Thomas Jefferson

Fitness—if it came in a bottle, everybody would have a great body.
Cher

There are two main types of exercise: aerobic and anaerobic. Aerobic exercise can be described as any activity that makes your heart beat faster and your rate of breathing increase: swimming, running, in-line skating, salsa dancing, skiing...you name it. Anaerobic exercise, or resistance training, refers to exercises like weight lifting.

Another way to think of these complementary forms of exercise is this: Aerobic exercise involves moving your entire body; anaerobic exercise usually involves remaining stationary while moving external weights. Both forms of exercise are associated with improved health outcomes. And when I say both, I mean doing both is better than doing only one or the other. If you're pressed for time, you can do aerobics one day and then anaerobic (resistance) exercise the next day. You don't need expensive equipment to do anaerobic exercises at home. This type of exercise can be done by using your own body weight (think push-ups, for example) or some inexpensive weights from a secondhand store.

For instance, studies have shown that the combination of resistance training and aerobics is the best possible strategy for improving insulin resistance and functional limitations in obese older people. Researchers controlled for other factors, such as age, sex and baseline insulin resistance values, and showed that subjects who engaged in both aerobics and strength training experienced greater improvements in insulin sensitivity and functional limitations than control subjects, who remained sedentary, or subjects who did only one form of exercise.

But if you can only manage one type—walking every day, for instance—then by all means, don't give up if you can't also fit in some weight training. It's always preferable to do *something* rather than nothing when it comes to exercise.

Simple walking is also an excellent form of exercise, especially for people with joint problems or for those who simply can't handle much physical activity initially. And while we're on the subject, I should mention that just about anything you do to get up and move can be counted towards your daily exercise goal.

Strategies to increase daily activity can include simple steps, like taking the stairs instead of the elevator, or parking as far from the door as possible, or owning a dog—which will need daily walks! People who work at desks should consider standing at least a few minutes each hour, if possible. Continuing to work while standing is one healthful new trend that seeks to address the inherent health risks of a desk job. The point is to get up and move! It's difficult to overemphasize this point. Think of it this way: Inactivity is toxic.

Relatively new research has deepened our realization of just how harmful inactivity can be. Sitting for hours on end at one's office desk, for example, contributes to weight gain and a flagging sense of energy. Here's a fascinating paradox: People who do not exercise are more likely to report feeling weary than people who get up off the couch and expend the energy to exercise.

It seems counterintuitive, but this has been demonstrated in experiments on human subjects. So the next time you reach for the "I'm too tired to exercise" excuse, remember this: *not* exercising makes you feel wearier than exercising would. Perhaps part of this effect is related to the cozy relationship between sleep and exercise. You need plenty of rest to engage in vigorous physical activity, and engaging in physical activity facilitates good sleep. This is what scientists call "positive synergy;" each improves the other. What's more, getting more sleep has been linked to better weight control.

According to research presented at an international conference on obesity, subjects who got a bad night's sleep ate 22% more than those who slept a full eight hours. Sleep-deprived subjects consumed an average of 550 more calories than subjects who got a full night of shut eye. Subjects who got just four hours of sleep reported feeling hungrier than subjects who slept eight hours.

The findings suggest that sleep deprivation promotes hunger. Of course, when people are hungry, they are more likely to overeat. For this reason, the study's presenters speculated that bad sleep habits may be contributing to the obesity epidemic.

Another study by Finnish researchers concluded that obesity is linked to poor sleep, even without sleep disturbances such as obstructive sleep apnea. Obstructive sleep apnea is a condition in which a person's excess weight affects the architecture of his airway, altering his ability to breathe properly while sleeping. Patients experience multiple awakenings each night as their breathing is interrupted. This interferes dramatically with the ability to cycle through all the regenerative phases of sleep, leaving sufferers tired, listless and sleep deprived. As you can see, sleep deprivation and obesity coexist in a vicious cycle.

It Helps Reduce Pain

Scientists at Norwegian University of Science and Technology reported not long ago that regular exercise reduces chronic pain. So pain is no excuse either. More than 46,000 Norwegians participated in the study. Turns out, the more people exercised, the less pain they experienced. On average, people ranging in age from 20 to 64 years reported up to 12% less pain with 30 minutes of moderate intensity exercise, one to three days per week. The prevalence of chronic pain among older women who exercised was even more dramatically reduced, by 21-38%, relative to women who did not exercise. To a lesser extent, this enhanced effect held true for older men as well.

What's surprising about the Norwegians' numbers is how large the benefit was relative to the time spent exercising. Some subjects did just 30 minutes per week, but even that was enough to make a difference. Of course, those who exercised more enjoyed even greater reductions in their chronic pain. But even a little helped!

This was underscored recently by Australian researchers, who studied the television viewing habits of older citizens and compared time spent in front of the tube (and on the couch) with viewers' health status. Guess what they found? Couch potatoes who spent the most time sitting were most likely to have symptoms of the metabolic syndrome. This is the obesity related condition that usually features three or more of the following conditions: high blood pressure, high blood sugar, abnormal blood lipids ("good" HDL too low; "bad" LDL too high; high triglycerides) and insulin resistance. People who reported spending the least time sitting in front of the TV had the lowest incidence of the metabolic syndrome.

Numerous studies have shown that engaging in regular exercise—and the weight loss that usually follows—is associated with better health outcomes among cancer survivors and people with autoimmune diseases, such as rheumatoid arthritis. Although rheumatoid arthritis can be a painful condition that would appear to limit a person's mobility, British scientists showed recently that patients who participated in "high-intensity progressive resistance training" (meaning they worked their muscles against incrementally greater amounts of weight) for six months lost weight and improved their mobility. These improvements remained in effect for up to three years after the end of the exercise program.

Committing to regular exercise doesn't have to be a distasteful chore. Just as switching to a more healthful diet needn't be viewed as a form of punishment, getting regular exercise can be fun. Most people I know who run every day, or swim laps every evening, or play tennis three times a week, do it because they love it, not because they feel obligated. Most of us love the result so much that we end up loving the whole process.

Lots of people don't particularly like working out initially, but after they start to experience the physical and mental benefits they find they love it, and actually look forward to it. I am one of them. That's the beauty of finding a form (or forms) of exercise that fits your lifestyle and preferences.

It can seem like a chore at first, and may require a measure of patience and perseverance on your part. But I can just about guarantee that eventually you'll find yourself looking forward to your daily exercise time. You'll realize how good it makes you feel, how much more energy you have, how your stress seems to dissolve with each step/stroke/push or pull, and how your mood lifts like a feather on the breeze. If it takes you outdoors, so much the better. Being outdoors is inherently therapeutic. Working out outdoors is a twofer, then.

A High Without Side-effects

The feelings of wellbeing induced by exercise have a basis in physiology. Scientists call it "exercise-induced euphoria" and note that this "runner's high" is at least partially due to the release of feel-good chemicals called beta-endorphins. These important chemicals help reduce stress, lower pain thresholds, and provide a sense of wellbeing.

Although you don't feel it at the time, they even boost immune system function and have been shown to slow the growth of cancer cells. Endorphins work by binding to target receptors, called opioid receptors, in the brain and nervous tissue. Not surprisingly, these are the same receptors targeted by plant-based opiates, such as opium and morphine. Of course, these drugs and their modern synthetic equivalents are used as powerful pain relievers in medicine. Despite the potency of these potentially addictive drugs, beta-endorphin is estimated to many times more potent as an analgesic than morphine.

But endorphins are not addictive, except in the sense described earlier: The more you exercise, and become accustomed to how good it makes you feel, the more you will want to continue exercising and experiencing that enhanced sense of wellbeing. The difference between the "high" obtained through exercise-induced endorphin release, and the artificial "high" of opioid drugs is that endorphins, which you must "earn," are nature's way of rewarding you for working your muscles and improving your fitness, while opiates taken as drugs of abuse are merely addictive and ultimately destructive.

Use It or Lose It

As the saying goes: "Use it or lose it." This cliché applies to muscle, certainly. If you don't work your muscles, they atrophy, losing mass and tone. But this inspirational slogan also applies to the rest of your body. In a sense, if you don't use "it" (your body) you may very well lose "it" (your health).

Technology has changed the amount of activity we once engaged in, allowing us to spend countless hours sitting in idle comfort. Problem is, all those modern conveniences that enable us to live lives of relative leisure have had unintended consequences, some of them serious.

From washing machines and automatic dryers to robotic vacuum cleaners and electric carts in grocery stores, our constant quest to eliminate drudgery has made life easier—and simultaneously more perilous. No one is suggesting that we abandon vacuum cleaners and go back to beating carpets outdoors each spring, but the point is that not every "improvement" that allows you to avoid physical activity is desirable.

There's simply no way around it: Our bodies remain dependent on physical activity to maintain optimal health and fitness. If you don't use "it" you'll lose far more than mere muscle mass. The cardiovascular system suffers, mood declines, energy flags, weight increases, and even your brain can start to lose mass. Talk about "use it or lose it!"

Inactivity is directly linked to obesity, and obesity is linked to a host of health woes, from increased risk of heart attack and stroke, to type 2 diabetes, to erectile dysfunction in men, to a greater risk of kidney disease, Alzheimer's disease, arthritis and other degenerative and inflammatory conditions.

Of course, it's somewhat easier to talk about exercise than it is to actually do it. Some of us make the effort, dutifully fitting in exercise on a regular basis, while others are probably tired of being reminded of the importance of exercise.

After all, it's so much easier to make excuses than to take action. We've all been there. I get it. I do. I'm a working mother myself. We tell ourselves, "I don't have enough time...I can't afford a gym membership...I don't like running...I have bad ankles/feet/knees (fill in the blank)...the weather's too hot (or too cold, or too wet)...My gym clothes are in the laundry...I hate to exercise...I'm already overstressed and overwhelmed," or my favorite: "I'm too tired." The list goes on and on.

I have a young son and a demanding career. I travel often and numerous people depend on me. There often seem to be too few hours in the day to accomplish all I need to do. As a physician, it's my job to know what ensures health and what foments disease. So I'm well aware of the importance of exercise. That's why I never take it for granted, and I almost never give in to the urge to fall back in bed for just a little more sleep at the expense of precious exercise time (don't get me wrong; adequate sleep is crucial for good health too. My solution: I go to bed early). The way I see it, my life is literally at stake.

Why Is It So Difficult?

I have found that lack of time and lack of habit are some of the biggest deterrents to regular exercise, especially for moms. I can tell you that's certainly the case for me! However, there is a solution. People don't always realize it, but any exercise is better than no exercise.

While it's true that a strenuous workout is great to increase your heart rate and release stress, it's also true that not everyone has thirty minutes to spare every day. As a working mother, I know that things like work, kids, laundry, meals, and appointments leave you with little time for yourself, especially when everyone at home wants a piece of you.

I've found that fitting in small workouts on a routine basis, combined with my True Nutrition plan can and will make a real difference in the way you feel and look. Exercise isn't only about health; it's also about self-esteem and a satisfying sense of accomplishment.

I say this as a woman and especially for my female readers: You deserve to feel good about yourself, and you deserve to have a bit of time for you. Why? It's simple. As I tell everyone at home, "Mom is a better mom when Mom has some *Mom time.*"

Have you ever felt totally sick of feeling not quite right? Perhaps your clothes don't look the way you want them to on your body, or your makeup doesn't seem to make you look the way you want, or every day becomes a bad-hair day, and nothing seems to go right. If this sounds familiar, believe me, I know how you feel. I've been there. And I've discovered that a mom who feels good about herself is a better mom, a better wife and a better employee.

Making Dreams Come True

The first step to achieving and maintaining a fitness regimen is to become determined. But your determination must be realistic. Start by working blocks of time into your schedule; write it down. Some women I've interviewed for this book say that exercise is difficult at the gym or at home.

If you're a working mother with small children, you have to get yourself and your children up even earlier than usual and take them to daycare at the health club, in order to get to the health club before work, and then take them to regular daycare before work. Needless to say, this adds to the guilt of leaving one's children in day care all day, and makes it even harder to get enough rest. Understandably, women in this situation are discouraged about getting to the gym on a regular basis.

For others, the idea of waking up even earlier is simply unattractive; I can also relate to that. Yet the message that I want to convey is that after you start exercising and seeing results in your own body, in the way you look and feel, you'll find that it gets easier. I'll talk more about schedules in a moment, but for now suffice it to say that having a written schedule makes things a lot easier. Workouts must be in your schedule, otherwise you will not do it. But if you have the dream of recovering your lost energy and getting back your body shape, determination will pay off.

Be Real, Not Ideal

We've all read reports claiming that you need to exercise for an hour or more, five or more days per week to really make a difference. Don't believe it. The truth is, any exercise is better than no exercise. So my first recommendation is this: Toss out the assumption that you have to exercise five or more hours a week to make an impact on your health and wellbeing. It's simply not true. Any amount of exercise you manage to squeeze into your schedule really does count. If you simply can't fit in a dedicated hour to workout every day, so be it. Don't let that discourage you from doing what you can. Yes, it would be ideal to be able to fit in a one-hour workout every day, but is it realistic?

If you think about our ancestors, you'll realize they didn't concern themselves with working out. The idea would probably have struck them as ludicrous, in fact. After all, who would have had the time? They were too busy going about the business of ordinary life; walking virtually everywhere, laboring on the land, toiling at their physically demanding jobs, lifting, loading, carrying, building, hauling water, cutting wood, and so on.

Unless they were householders with servants, even the women worked hard, doing by hand everything we now do with convenient machines. These hard-working folks also consumed wholesome, healthful foods. Refined sugars and processed foods were virtually nonexistent. These days our lives have changed drastically. Sugar is cheap and abundant. We've already talked about the dangers of sugar. Far from being a rare and expensive treat, it is virtually everywhere.

We've also become far more sedentary than our ancestors, toiling at desks rather than behind plows; sitting in cars rather than walking or riding horses; turning a tap handle, rather than hauling a heavy bucket or working a pump handle. We're also exposed to more insidious environmental toxins, many of which never existed before. Mankind has always faced exposure to certain toxins, whether from the natural environment, or resulting from industry, but many modern chemicals are something new. Many are subtle, and extremely widespread. And unlike, say, coal dust, they tend to be invisible.

Clearly, we need to actively pursue exercise to keep our bodies healthy, in a way that our ancestors never needed to consider. While technology has provided marvelous conveniences and astonishing advances that have given us ever-more leisure time, the human body has not changed. It's still designed for physical activity, on a daily basis. Without getting up and moving, our bodies quickly become weak and susceptible to illness. This has been demonstrated again and again. Sitting is literally toxic, while moving is tonic. It's just that simple.

If fitting exercise into your schedule is daunting, perhaps it would help to break it up a bit. So instead of planning to exercise for an hour a day, why not plan for thirty minutes, or for two blocks of fifteen minutes each, one in the morning, one in the evening? Or even three blocks of ten minutes each? If you overdo it, you're more likely to get burned out, which makes it easier to justify giving up. And that's counterproductive. Simply strive to do more than you've been doing, even if it's just a little more. Increase the length or intensity of your workouts gradually.

And that will put you on your way to a healthier you. By reading this book and taking charge of your own body you are doing yourself a favor. Follow my True Nutrition Plan for Vibrant Health, and include a reasonable amount of exercise, and you will start to feel a difference in your life. You'll also make a difference in your long-term health outlook.

The Schedule

Someone once said, "The key is not to prioritize what's on your schedule, but to schedule your priorities." Not all successful people live on a tight schedule, but having a good schedule can make you even more successful. If you *don't* love exercise, it's even more important that you add exercise time to your agenda.

I know people who think a mental calendar is good enough. I strongly disagree. To succeed with my program you are going to need a written calendar. Use a computer or write by hand. After analyzing your personal situation and deciding what days you can exercise and for how long, enter it in the system or write it on the calendar filling that time slot with "exercise". Print several copies and post them in different areas of your house, so you can see your schedule regularly. Keep one near your computer, in the kitchen, and in the bathroom. These small reminders work wonders to help you achieve your dream. I promise.

I exercise daily, but have not set foot in a health club for more than a decade.

Secrets to remember:

- Any activity is better than no activity.
- Be realistic about what you can do.
- Once you experience the physical reward of regular exercise it will become easier.

To find out what exercises I recommend, and how to fit them into your busy life, visit my website at CocoMarch.com. Download a free "how to" report by entering the key words: "Skip the Gym."

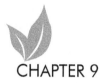

CHAPTER 9

Transitioning

*To keep the body in good health is a duty, otherwise we
shall not be able to keep our mind strong and clear.*
Buddha

*Hunger and thirst scarcely kill any,
but gluttony and drink kill a great many.*
Latin proverb

B y now we've learned about some of the unexpected places where toxic chemicals lurk, and why you should avoid them. We've discussed why eating organic meats, dairy, fruits and vegetables may help you reduce your risk of various health conditions. And we've covered the dangers you are exposing your body to when consuming excess sugars. Now we're ready to put it all into practice and begin the transition process.

In sports, transitioning refers to changes made when shifting from defense to offense, or from offense to defense. I learned this from my husband Mike, who loves every sport known to man. Although I don't necessarily appreciate how challenging transitioning can be in the context of sports, I can relate to it when it comes to transitioning from a non-nutritious lifestyle to a True Nutrition lifestyle.

Dr. Cocó's True Nutrition avoids the pitfalls of the typical American diet. I am giving you the tools you need to succeed, including my True Nutrition recipes, which are quick and easy to make. Download them for free at CocoMarch.com by entering the key word "recipes." You can also explore and create your own recipes. Just make sure your meals consist of more plants, grains, and legumes, and perhaps a little less meat. The nutrients from my meals encourage a lifestyle featuring the benefits of veganism combined with the pleasures of eating realistic amounts of meat, fish and dairy.

Dr. Cocó's 10 True Secrets

Step One: Increase your plant consumption at every meal; boost your intake of antioxidants.

Step Two: Focus on eating whole foods rather than packaged foods; eliminate unnatural chemicals.

Step Three: Replace less healthy options with healthier ones; even small changes can add up to big benefits.

Step Four: Find time to be physically active.

Step Five: Meals should consist of a balanced combination of proteins, fats and carbohydrates.

Step Six: Switch to smaller plates and bowls.

Step Seven: Be aware of food portions.

Step Eight: Do not count calories.

Step Nine: Do not skip meals.

Step Ten: Enjoy some red wine.

To better effect change, it helps to understand why these dietary and lifestyle changes are beneficial. We've already seen that many common toxins pose a threat to health. But how do whole foods benefit us? I think of them as health insurance. Like an insurance policy, eating whole foods is an investment in the future. You may not reap noticeable benefits immediately. But just as toxins, chemicals, or junk food don't kill you overnight, healthy food doesn't heal suddenly; it happens gradually. But trust me, it happens.

Antioxidants and Free Radicals

Antioxidants are substances found in large amounts in fruits, vegetables, nuts, spices, legumes and whole grains. They're substances that help protect your body's cells from damage that can be caused by free radicals. The more antioxidants available in your body, the greater your overall defense against the diseases associated with free radical damage.

The term *free radical* has been in fairly common use for decades now, but from talking to people I've come to realize that many folks have only the vaguest understanding of what a free radical is and what it does. Someone once told me, "It's just too technical a concept for me to understand." I understand her position, but I think it's helpful to have a mental image of what these reactive molecules are, to appreciate why neutralizing free radicals is so beneficial.

Free Radicals Made Simple

Free radicals have been associated with tissue damage in our bodies and many researchers believe they are the culprits behind numerous degenerative diseases, such as Alzheimer's, or even certain cancers. Free radical damage can occur from exposure to certain chemicals, smoking, pollution, radiation, and even as a byproduct of normal metabolism. In other words, we are *all* exposed to this damage. The key, therefore, is to create a protective barrier against these reactive molecules, in a manner of speaking.

Free radicals are molecules that are missing one electron. To survive, these "incomplete" molecules steal from other molecules to satisfy their "need" for the missing electron. Unfortunately, the cannibalized molecule becomes a free radical in turn.

Let's pretend you and your feet are molecules, and your shoes are electrons. Imagine you are a free radical, so you're going about your daily business with a missing shoe. You have work to do and miles to travel, but you're hobbled by having only one shoe. It's awkward and painful to walk, but you have to keep moving. You are ruthless, and you're desperate for relief. You see another traveler walking along, smiling, wearing *two* shoes. In your size. You grab a shoe off the traveler as he passes, and put it on your own bare foot. Now you can walk with ease. But the hapless traveler whom you stole from is now hobbling down the road, unbalanced and uncomfortable. He's now desperate to steal a replacement shoe. His fellow travelers had better look out. And so the cycle will continue.

This process happens millions of times each day in our bodies. If these dangerous free radicals are not stabilized they create a vicious cycle of stealing electrons from healthy molecules, and turning those molecules into new free radicals which in turn have to steal more electrons from other molecules. To extend our analogy, imagine millions of people stumbling around stealing shoes from each other, every minute of every day.

Stopping the Cycle

Antioxidants are important because they have *extra* electrons; they act as electron donors. Using the shoe analogy again, imagine a person traveling among all the crippled people stumbling about on one shoe. This person, let's call her Auntie Oxidant, is freely dispensing shoes (one size fit all!) to anyone stumbling along on one shoe. Stabilized by having two sturdy shoes, the formerly crippled people are able to return to work at full efficiency.

Antioxidants possess spare electrons. When they encounter a free radical with a missing electron, they freely donate an electron to help stabilize the needy molecule. No harm is done, because as a donor molecule, the antioxidant also remains stable. The free radical gets the electron it needs to become stable, so it doesn't need to steal from another molecule. The cycle of theft is broken and other cells are free to go about their business.

Free radicals can be created through exposure to pesticides, pollution, stress, radiation (such as X-rays) and other triggers. The higher one's free radical count, the more important it becomes to have a sufficient supply of antioxidants in the body, to help keep them in check.

Hari Sharma, M.D., in his book *Freedom from Disease* notes that pesticides, and even some preservatives used in foods, kill unwanted "pests" by overwhelming their defenses with free radicals. Problem is, he says, when we consume these free radicals they accumulate in our bodies and eventually harm us, too.

Free radicals can come from just about anywhere: automobile exhaust, meat in the diet, even mental stress. Any of these can lead to overproduction of free radicals in the body. Free radicals will attack any type of molecule to obtain a missing electron, but it takes different types of antioxidants to most efficiently neutralize free radicals among different type of cells. As you can see, it's crucial to increase one's intake of natural antioxidants from fresh fruits and vegetables, as well as to eat a variety of them.

The Protective Role of Antioxidants

To better understand how much antioxidants can protect our bodies from the inside out, consider what happens when you slice an apple. If left exposed to air, the fruit will eventually turn brown. This is due to oxidation that occurs when the fruit's cells interact with oxygen in the air.

The same process of oxidation occurs inside our bodies at the cellular level. Damage can be caused by free radicals produced by environmental factors, as I mentioned earlier: pollution, radiation, cigarette smoke, herbicides, pesticides, the wrong foods, stress, and more. Think again of the apple slice, exposed to air and quickly turning brown. As any savvy cook knows, if you drizzle some lemon juice on it, it will remain temptingly white. That's because lemon juice is high in antioxidants, such as ascorbic acid (vitamin C), and bioflavonoids. Try this at home if you've never experienced this simple chemistry experiment. It provides a graphic illustration of the protective properties of natural antioxidants in food.

Oxidation occurs millions of times daily within our bodies. Some oxidation is beneficial; without it we could not extract sufficient energy from our food. But runaway oxidative processes, as we've seen, can also encourage disease. This "oxidative stress" can be slowed down dramatically when our bodies have a large supply of healthy antioxidants. Just as lemon juice splashed on a cut apple preserves the apple's appeal, a rich supply of antioxidants in the bloodstream slows the internal oxidation of cells, lowering the risk of heart disease, infection and perhaps even some forms of cancer.

Organic Versus Conventionally Grown

I mentioned before that common pesticides, herbicides and other chemicals used in today's agriculture industry are not only dangerous, but they also create free radicals. The amount of man-made pesticides used to grow most produce is alarming. Likewise, the endless quantities of antibiotics and hormones that are forced on conventionally raised animals is more than a little concerning. When we eat meat raised in this manner, these chemicals end up in our own bodies, where they are stored in our fatty tissues. And that detracts from vibrant health and wellness.

Certainly no one would want to apply man-made pesticides directly to the skin, as one might do with a paste made from turmeric root in India, to improve one's complexion, or to heal a wound. On the contrary, accidental skin exposure to man-made pesticides is a significant route by which agricultural workers are poisoned by these dangerous chemicals. Just working with them requires extensive precautions, including the wearing of masks, protective clothing and gloves. As consumers, we are routinely assured that these unnatural chemicals are perfectly safe, but common sense tells us otherwise.

The fact remains that pesticides used in agriculture—primarily a class of chemicals known as organophosphates—are toxic not only to insects, but also to humans. Granted, they pose a recognized risk only at higher doses, and agribusiness claims that pesticide residue levels are negligible in table-ready food.

It is troubling that these "safe" chemicals have been associated with symptoms that include headache, dizziness, fatigue, nausea, breathing problems, abdominal cramps and tingling in the extremities. These symptoms have been reported in adults working with pesticides and in children living nearby who were inadvertently exposed to them, primarily through drift from crop-dusting.

Scientists in Israel studied this problem on collective farms called kibbutzim, in the early 1990s. Affected individuals experienced decreased rates of nerve conduction, indicating that exposure resulted in some level of neurological insult. Other studies have shown that pesticide exposure may be also be related to an elevated risk of developing certain cancers, as well neurological, mental and reproductive effects.

There are at least 40 different organophosphate pesticides in use in the United States, and about 73 million pounds of these nervous system disruptors are released into the environment every year. This is alarming, when you consider that this chemical class includes nerve gas agents, such as sarin and VX nerve agent.

Organophosphates can enter the body through multiple routes, including absorption through the skin, inhalation and ingestion. While most of us are extremely unlikely to be accidentally exposed directly, the Israeli experience serves to illustrate the dangers of over-exposure. Workers were clearly exposed to unsafe levels of these toxins. But who is to say what level of a nerve toxin is truly "safe"? Scientists routinely assess the lethal effects of any given toxin, and formulate guidelines regarding presumptive safe levels of exposure. If risk increases with exposure, and exposure is cumulative, isn't it best to avoid these harmful chemicals, if at all possible?

Pesticides and Children

Unfortunately, children are most at risk from pesticide exposure, due to a variety of factors. For one, their natural detoxification pathways (primarily in the liver) are often underdeveloped compared to those of adults. For another, they live longer, so diseases such as cancer, which may be triggered over long periods of time, have longer to manifest.

Most recently, scientists announced that pesticides pose an especially high risk to developing fetuses. A pregnant woman who comes into contact with even common household pesticides may risk endangering her developing fetus, at a time when her fetus is most vulnerable. For these reasons, I trust in buying and serving organic produce whenever possible. I know it's more expensive, and it may be challenging to find adequate organic produce where you live. But in a world where any number of formerly rare diseases is on the rise, I can't help but think it's the least we can do to protect our health and that of our families.

Transitioning to Organic

Obviously, one of the primary advantages of buying organic is that you avoid exposure to pesticides, which are used extensively to grow "conventional" crops. I have to confess I didn't always buy all organic. I always bought organically raised meats, but it wasn't until I investigated and found more research supporting the dangers of pesticides, that I made the decision to switch to 100% organically grown produce and plant-based natural soaps and cleaners. Given all I'd learned, the choice was clear. I knew I had to make the switch.

Implementing these seemingly simple changes was less than simple, though. In fact, at first it seemed overwhelming. There are so many options that evaluating them all and choosing the ones that work best for your family can be daunting. I know it was for me.

I quickly discovered that most organic foods are about 30% more expensive than conventionally grown foods. Depending on where you live, your options for shopping at organic grocery stores that offer a wide range of organic foods may range from excellent to non-existent. West coast states like California, Oregon and Washington State seem to offer a broad variety of organic stores. But other states tend to be a bit more problematic, with a more conservative selection of organic foods.

While organic fruits, vegetables and meats are produced without the use of pesticides, antibiotics and hormones, they also do not contain any added preservatives. So their shelf life is often less than that of nonorganic foods. This means that you may need to buy your fresh fruits and vegetables more than once a week. I know this can be more challenging, but if you keep everything in the fridge, as opposed to sitting on the counter, you can extend the shelf life of these products by a few more days.

At times buying everything organic is simply not possible. Maybe you can't afford to convert to buying 100% organic groceries. But you can start by avoiding the foods with the highest amounts of pesticides, according to the following list. When in doubt about produce, keep the following rule of thumb in mind: Fruits and vegetables with thicker skins tend to contain fewer pesticides.

These are guidelines published by the Environmental Working Group, a non-profit consumer safety organization. According to EWG, these are the top common foods that are most and least likely to contain problematic levels of pesticides. EWG publishes a new list annually; some details may change.

Highest in pesticides	Lowest in pesticides
Celery	Onions
Peaches	Avocados
Strawberries	Sweet Corn
Apples	Pineapple
Blueberries	Mangos
Nectarines	Sweet Peas
Bell Peppers	Asparagus
Spinach	Kiwi
Cherries	Cabbage
Kale/Collard Greens	Eggplant
Potatoes	Cantaloupe
Grapes (imported)	Watermelon
	Grapefruit
	Sweet Potato
	Honeydew Melon

It's becoming increasingly common for local grocery stores to have an organic section where you can find a lot of certified organic fruits, vegetables and meats, but I want to provide a few guidelines if you are just getting started.

Strategic Moves

If you are frugal like me, with a family to feed, you may want to visit stores like Costco and Trader Joe's. They offer many organically grown foods at competitive prices. Not everything they carry is organic, though, so keep an eye on what you are buying. Keep in mind that "100% natural" is not the same as organic in most cases.

The term "all natural" may be misleading. A 100% natural pre-made lasagna will most likely be made with cheese and ground beef from cows raised eating corn instead of grass. The cows may have been treated with antibiotics and hormones, and the tomatoes may have been grown with pesticides and herbicides. Meanwhile, the pasta may be made from wheat that is genetically modified.

The term "all natural" can be misleading because it simply means that the manufacturer did not add chemicals to the final product. So even though the ingredients may contain pesticides, herbicides, antibiotics or hormones, no additional preservatives have been added to the final product. As you can see, despite the "all natural" label, the reality is not as simple as the term implies.

 ## Secrets to remember:

- Increase the variety of fruits and vegetables you eat every day.
- Start buying produce and other products from local farmers (as long as they raise them without chemicals), or buy them organic.
- If you can't afford to buy everything organic, avoid the produce that has been found to contain the highest amounts of pesticides.
- Do not purchase items labeled "all natural" or "100% natural". Most likely they contain pesticides, herbicides, antibiotics or hormones.

Want easy tips on how to transition to organic while staying within your budget? Visit my website CocoMarch.com. Enter the key words "Organic Budget" and download my free report.

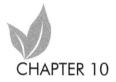

CHAPTER 10

Powerhouse Nutrients

Nothing will benefit human health and increase the chances for
survival of life on Earth as much as the evolution to a vegetarian diet.
Albert Einstein

Trueue Nutrition is a whole food diet; I endorse a lifestyle that provides the benefits of a diet rich in fiber, natural oils, fruits, vegetables, grains, seeds, and some lean meats and dairy. Why are we encouraged to eat a diet rich in fiber and essential fats? Why are fruits and vegetables always part of what is called a healthy lifestyle? Why can't we skip those foods, if we choose? To answer this question, let's take a closer look at phytonutrients.

Phytonutrients—literally, nutrients from plants—include many unique substances with remarkably beneficial properties. For the most part, these are chemical compounds that a plant manufactures for its own benefit. When we consume these plants, we share in the benefits.

Our relationship with plants has insured that these remarkable substances work with our bodies on a molecular level, in often astoundingly elegant ways, to promote health. So part of the problem is that too many people eat too few plant foods, and get too few crucial nutrients as a result. In addition to phytonutrients, plants and grains also provide fiber.

It Could Save Your Life

What's the big deal about fiber? A randomized study published in the *Archives of Internal Medicine* showed that dietary fiber is effective at reducing levels of C-reactive protein (CRP). C-reactive protein is an inflammatory marker associated with the development and progression of various inflammatory, lifestyle-related common diseases, such as diabetes, atherosclerosis and an increased risk of cardiovascular disease.

Subjects represented a wide range of ages, body types and ethnicities, including lean and obese, black and white, and younger and older individuals. Led by investigators at the Medical University of South Carolina, the study clearly showed that a higher fiber intake of about 30 grams a day can reduce CRP levels. It made no difference whether the higher intake of fiber came from a diet naturally rich in fiber, or from supplements.

One of the less obvious benefits of eating a near-vegetarian diet, such as the Mediterranean diet, or the Dietary Approaches to Stop Hypertension (DASH) diet, is the abundance of natural plant-based fiber that these diets deliver. A higher fiber intake is associated with a number of health benefits, including a significantly reduced risk of developing colorectal cancer, for starters. It also helps reduce chronic inflammation. Left unchecked, chronic inflammation may lead to the development of a number of serious conditions.

The benefits of whole-grain oats are even better than scientists originally believed, according to pioneering researchers. A decade after the U.S. Food and Drug Administration noted that consumption of oatmeal may reduce the risk of coronary heart disease, and granted manufacturers the right to make an initial "heart-healthy" claim for oats, investigators published another report in the *American Journal of Lifestyle Medicine*, again extolling the virtues of oats and their remarkable fiber benefits.

The newer research shows that the consumption of oats and oat products significantly reduces total cholesterol and LDL-cholesterol concentrations, without adversely affecting HDL-cholesterol or triglyceride levels. Even better, the new data show that when oats are included in a lifestyle-management program, they provide additional health benefits that may go beyond mere cholesterol control. These benefits include a decreased tendency towards obesity, a reduced risk of diabetes, and the possibility that oats may reduce the risk of atherosclerosis.

Fiber and You

True Nutrition—with its emphasis on fresh, unprocessed vegetables, fruits, grains, and nuts—supplies the vitamins, minerals, and trace elements that help protect us from oxidative damage and inflammation. It also supplies far more fiber than the average American diet contains. This is no small point. Emerging evidence suggests that fiber is an often overlooked, highly underrated component of a healthful diet.

The truth is, people who eat fiber-rich diets (especially fiber from whole grains) live longer than those who don't, according to the results of a recently published study. That's why I encourage you to replace polished or processed white grains with whole grains. Choose brown rice over white rice, for instance. Substitute whole wheat products for foods made with refined white flour.

Previous studies have linked higher fiber consumption to a lower risk of heart disease, diabetes, high blood pressure, breast cancer and colon cancer. The latest research, sponsored in part by the National Institutes of Health, is believed to be the first to clearly show that eating more fiber translates to longer overall lifespan. It's been estimated that the average American gets just 9-11 g of fiber per day, despite the fact that adults should get 25-38 g of fiber per day.

But what about fat, should we avoid it or embrace it?

Fat Is Not a Four-letter Word

Too much fat of any kind is undesirable. As in most things, moderation is key. It's true that fat molecules pack more calories—more available energy—per unit of weight than carbohydrates or proteins. So an ounce of fat has inherently more calories than an ounce of protein, for example.

But we need both for good health and adequate nutrition. So fat is not "evil," per se. But not all fats are created equal. Some are relatively good and some are decidedly bad. As we've already discussed, saturated fat, and especially trans fats, probably do more harm than good to the body. In contrast, polyunsaturated and monounsaturated fats, found primarily in plant foods, are actually good for the heart and blood vessels. Trans fats should be avoided at all costs; they are, in essence, poison to a healthy cardiovascular system.

Here's the take-home message: Fats from most plants are healthful. Avocados are an example of a plant-based food that is very high in fat content, while still being good for you. It is packed with monounsaturated fat and vitamin E, and provides some fiber and other nutrients.

Walnuts are another example of a high-fat, heart-healthy food. They are one of the few plant sources of the omega-3 fatty acid, ALA, which is converted in the body into DHA (docosahexaenoic acid) and EPA (eicosapentaenoic acid). Of course, these anti-inflammatory and heart-healthy omega-3 fatty acids are crucial for vibrant health, as they are essential nutrients.

Where Have All the (Good) Fatty Acids Gone?

By now most people have heard about omega-3 fatty acids. These "good" fats, found primarily in cold water fish—and to a lesser extent in plant foods such as flaxseed and walnuts—are nutritional headliners because an increased intake of omega-3s is associated with a slew of health benefits.

Omega-3s are considered essential fatty acids. Essential nutrients are substances that the body absolutely requires for proper functioning, but cannot manufacture internally. I think it's extremely important to note that modern Western diets have shifted so far from consumption of omega-3s towards intake of omega-6s that this ratio is now estimated to be about 25:1.

And that's a big problem. At the risk of oversimplification, omega-6 fatty acids are converted in the body to pro-inflammatory (inflammation-promoting) compounds, while omega-3 fatty acids play the opposite role, supplying building blocks for a number of anti-inflammatory compounds.

As you might imagine, when these two nutrients and their derivatives are in balance, the body is better able to balance the need for inflammation (to promote infection fighting, for instance) with anti-inflammatory activity, when it's time to put out the flames and allow things to calm back down.

The benefits of having a diet rich in omega-3 fatty acids range from a lower risk of depression, heart disease, and cancer, to better mood and a decreased risk of arthritis and other inflammatory diseases. If our Western diets had not changed so dramatically in the past few generations, we probably wouldn't be talking about omega-3s as nutritional superstars. Omega-3s certainly are some of the most remarkable, beneficial nutrients we can add to the diet to achieve better overall health. But that's because most of us are still eating far too few of these nutrients, while consuming far too many of their chemical cousins, the omega-6 fatty acids.

Past generations consumed a diet richer in essential fatty acids. For instance, alpha-linolenic acid (ALA), comes from plant sources. Our bodies can convert ALA into the other omega-3s we need. In his book "Supplements Exposed," Brian R. Clement, PhD notes that plenty of plants provide beneficial omega-3s, including chia seeds, raspberry seeds, pumpkin seeds, walnuts, hemp seeds, flax seeds, sprouts, algae and dark green leafy vegetables, such as kale and spinach. These foods were consumed much more often by our ancestors, hence the emphasis on including such power nutrients in our daily lives.

Omega-3-fatty acids are also abundant in fatty cold-water fish, such as salmon, tuna and sardines. Omega-3s are crucial for good health. These essential nutrients have been shown to reduce levels of triglycerides in the blood and to decrease the incidence of depression and inflammation, among other benefits. A high level of triglycerides—a condition called hypertriglyceridemia—is another factor contributing to the metabolic syndrome and an elevated risk of diabetes and heart disease.

As I mentioned earlier, fish can be a generous source of these precious fatty acids. The sad news is that much commercially available fish, even when wild-caught, can be polluted with heavy metals such as mercury and lead. The other option is farm-raised fish, but Dr. Clement notes that this is not always better. Some farm-raised fish contains even higher levels of toxins than fish caught in the wild. Some of this is due to aquaculture practices that include feeding ground-up fishmeal to captive fish. Problem is, the fishmeal may be made from fish already contaminated with toxins.

Unnaturally crowded conditions force farmers to feed antibiotics to farm-raised fish, to avoid rampant infections.

So where does that leave us to obtain the omega-3 fatty acids we need? I recommend plant-based omega-3s, or if you choose fish oil, purchase molecularly distilled omega-3s from a reliable source. Heavy metals have been removed from these products. These distilled oils are usually tested to ensure they are free of potentially harmful levels of contaminants (i.e. mercury, heavy metals, PCBs, dioxins, and other contaminants) while still providing omega-3 essential fatty acids.

Does that mean that you should never eat fish? Some people would argue that if you know something may contain toxins, you should stay as far away from it as possible. Ideally, this makes sense. But we're focusing on being real, instead of ideal. Accordingly, I believe it's more practical to advise eating fish in moderation. In short, I think the benefits of consuming fish outweigh the risks.

However, if you are pregnant or nursing, check with your doctor. He or she can advise you regarding which fish is best, and which should be avoided. As a rule of thumb, larger predatory species tend to have higher levels of mercury, due to a process called bioaccumulation, in which mercury becomes concentrated as bigger fish eat smaller fish, and so on.

Vitamin C

Vitamin C is another essential nutrient, commonly found in fresh fruits and vegetables. It has occasionally been promoted as something of a wonder drug. While it won't cure everything, it is a potent natural antioxidant widely available in nature. We have already discussed the dramatic benefits of a diet rich in antioxidants to help reduce free radical damage, which may help avert an array of diseases while reducing the risk of certain cancers. Vitamin C is also a cofactor necessary for a number of enzymatic reactions.

Studies have shown that low levels of vitamin C are linked to an increased prevalence of cardiovascular and kidney disease. Vitamin C is believed to play a role in protecting the lining of the blood vessels from dysfunction by reducing oxidative stress, thereby protecting against the development of atherosclerosis and kidney disease alike. Vitamin C is readily available from a good diet, such as the Mediterranean diet, but supplementation is considered safe, if desired.

In 2011, European scientists published some results from a large, long-term study, which examined the relationship between blood pressure and plasma levels of vitamin C (from fruits and vegetables in the diet). People with the highest concentrations of vitamin C were 22% less likely to have high blood pressure, even after accounting for other possible factors that might also affect blood pressure, such as age, sex, body mass index, smoking, etc. The authors offered the findings as further evidence of an apparent strong link between high fruit and vegetable intake (and higher intake of vitamin C) and healthier, lower blood pressure.

Another recent study concluded that supplementation with an average of 500 milligrams of vitamin C per day is linked to a significant reduction in uric acid levels in the bloodstream. This is another very good thing: High uric acid levels are strongly linked to painful and potentially debilitating gout. This Medieval-sounding ailment, which manifests as excruciating pain in the joints, is increasingly common. The pain is caused by the formation of sharp crystals in the joints—crystals of pure uric acid.

The study was a meta-analysis; a type of study that incorporates data from other previously published studies on the subject. In this case, the included studies were all randomized, controlled trials—considered the highest standard when it comes to drawing conclusions about the effects of a specific nutrient on human health.

The North American Dietary Reference Intake recommends that adults get about 60 to 90 mg of vitamin C daily. But up to 500 mg (one-half gram) per day is considered safe, and even higher amounts are unlikely to do harm.

Include in your diet high-vitamin C foods like strawberries, acerola cherries, oranges, grapefruits, lemons, limes, papayas, blackcurrant, kiwi, bell peppers, brussels sprouts, cantaloupe, kale, mustard greens, spinach, broccoli, cauliflower, tomatoes and even herbs such as cilantro and parsley.

Following this advice will provide you with plenty of naturally occurring full spectrum vitamin C. Natural vitamin C usually occurs with other nutrients called bioflavonoids, which your body uses to better absorb it. For instance, vitamin C from citrus fruits is more effective than synthetic vitamin C you may purchase at the store. Just eat a plethora of the above fruits and vegetables and you will obtain plenty of vitamin C

Vitamin D

Let's explore the concept of essential nutrients a little more deeply. We'll take the example of vitamin D, another essential nutrient. It's also gained increased attention in recent years, owing to two emerging sets of information. First, we have only recently begun to appreciate just how versatile, ubiquitous and crucial this hormone-like vitamin is, and just how far-reaching its impact on numerous aspects of health and well being.

Second, in recent years scientists have carefully documented people's blood levels of vitamin D, and the results are disturbing. It turns out the vast majority of us spend most of our time in a state of vitamin D insufficiency or deficiency, according to these studies. This is a concern because vitamin D is so crucial for health. Its effects go far beyond merely insuring strong bones.

In fact, it's so crucial it's one of the few essential nutrients that we are capable of producing internally. This eliminates the need to rely on dietary sources, and should ensure that we always have a ready supply. By harnessing the power of sunlight falling on bare skin, the body is able to convert common, readily available molecules circulating in the bloodstream into a vitamin D precursor molecule.

This precursor must undergo further transformation before it is released into the circulation as the active form of the vitamin. This elaborate mechanism evolved because vitamin D is one of the most important hormones in the body. As evidence of this, we need only consider the distribution of receptors for this molecule. They are located on virtually every tissue, in every organ (including the brain), throughout the body. By engaging with these receptors, like a key in a lock, vitamin D helps regulate countless functions, including immunity. In recent years, scientists have begun to more fully appreciate the tremendous importance of adequate levels of vitamin D for overall health and wellness.

One interesting study examined the birth and medical records of more than six million children born in California between 1990 and 2002. Investigators wondered if the time of a child's conception or birth might have any influence on his or her relative risk of developing autism. Interestingly, babies conceived in the winter months of December, January, and February had a 6% greater risk of subsequently being diagnosed with autism before their sixth birthday, compared with children conceived in summer. The researchers suggested that this might represent a seasonally variable environmental cause for autism.

While they did not offer any speculations about the possible identity of this variable, I think it's suspicious that vitamin D levels are known to fall dramatically during the winter months in North America. Given that vitamin D receptors are located on virtually every type of tissue in the human body, including brain cells, it seems at least plausible that vitamin D deficiency or insufficiency among pregnant mothers may play some small but not insignificant role as a risk factor for autism spectrum disorders (ASD).

This speculation takes on added weight when considered in the context of another new study, which found that a high proportion of newborns and their mothers in the Boston area were vitamin D deficient. Even among women taking prenatal vitamins, investigators found, more than 30% were vitamin D insufficient. The amount of supplemental vitamin D provided by the prenatal vitamins was evidently too little to boost mothers' blood levels into the ideal range.

Another recent study found widespread vitamin D insufficiency among pregnant women living in the Deep South, despite the lower latitude, where the sun's ultraviolet rays are stronger for a longer portion of the year. Investigators noted that African-American and Hispanic women were especially likely to have insufficient or even deficient levels of the "sunshine vitamin."

Dr. John Cannell, founder of the nonprofit Vitamin D Council, which promotes vitamin D awareness, has stated that vitamin D is probably crucial to brain development, protecting brain cells and helping them grow. "In addition," says Dr. Cannell, "autism is likely mediated by inflammation, and vitamin D is a key player in anti-inflammatory processes."

Of course, only time and further study will reveal the true causes of this heartbreaking spectrum of disorders, but this would not be the first condition linked to vitamin D insufficiency or deficiency. In recent years, numerous studies have shown that vitamin D levels have fallen precipitously among Americans in the past few generations.

This is probably related to a combination of factors. Vitamin D is generated naturally when sunlight strikes bare skin in summer. But our modern lifestyles have conspired to drastically impede this process. We have been conditioned to slavishly apply sunscreen whenever exposure to sunlight is anticipated, we spend more time indoors than our forebears (due, in no small part to the widespread use of air conditioning in both cars and buildings), and children are even less likely to spend time playing outdoors than they did in previous generations.

Public policy makers have been slow to adapt to rapidly accumulating new information about the importance of adequate vitamin D levels. This tsunami of new research indicates that vitamin D is crucial for everything from healthy immune system function, to cardiovascular disease prevention, to cancer prevention, to mood regulation and beyond. In fact, in 2010 the Institute of Medicine (an independent arm of the National Academy of Sciences) finally moved to modestly raise recommendations regarding adequate daily intake of vitamin D for adults and children. The change came after years of strenuous insistence by experts in the field that the former recommendations were set too low.

Former intake guidelines were based on limited data regarding the amount of vitamin D required to prevent rickets, a bone disease that represents the most extreme outcome of severe vitamin D deficiency. But thousands of new studies over the past few decades have consistently shown that vitamin D plays a far more important and complex role in maintaining health than was previously known. Bone health is only the tip of the iceberg, so to speak, when it comes to this amazing vitamin-like hormone. Some experts believe that the new guidelines issued by the Institute of Medicine are still too modest to achieve the full potential benefits of higher blood levels of vitamin D.

Secrets to remember:

- A healthful diet includes plenty of whole foods.
- Many Americans do not get enough fiber. Don't be one of them.
- Certain essential nutrients, such as vitamin C and omega-3 fatty acids, must be obtained through the diet, or, in the case of vitamin D, through sensible sun exposure and/or supplementation.
- Consider supplementing with fish oil to get enough heart-healthy omega-3 fatty acids into your diet.

CHAPTER 11

A Mediterranean Tale

O Love! what hours were thine and mine,
In lands of palm and southern pine;
In lands of palm, of orange blossom,
Of olive, aloe, and maize and vine!
Alfred, Lord Tennyson

The story of the Mediterranean diet probably began in the Fertile Crescent bordering the eastern Mediterranean Sea many thousands of years ago. The people who lived and farmed the region benefited handsomely from the illustrious Mediterranean climate; a specific combination of rainfall, moderate temperature and reliable sunshine that supports a variety of healthful foodstuffs, including olives, grapes, pomegranates, dates, grains, aromatic herbs and other plants.

These people lived simply; working the land, tending goats and sheep, and gathering seafood from the bountiful sea. The region features various populations with diverse customs, languages, political structures and beliefs, but a similar diet united them all in robust health.

The modern world got its first inkling of the special health benefits of the Mediterranean diet soon after World War II. Physiologist

Ancel Keys spent time in Spain after being stationed in Italy. He grew interested in the traditional cuisines of the area and eventually met fellow scientists from the region who were studying the dietary habits of various local populations.

In time, Keys published reports on the famous Seven Countries Study, a landmark scientific investigation of locals' dietary habits, which filtered into the public consciousness in the early 1970s. American deaths from heart disease had reached an alarming peak in the 1960s, and scientists had only recently begun to understand the link between blood cholesterol levels and cardiovascular health.

A key finding of the studies revealed that certain Mediterranean populations possessed extraordinarily low cholesterol levels, while also enjoying a remarkably low incidence of heart disease and cancer. Only later did scientists discern that cholesterol is only part of the story. Inflammation and oxidative stress caused by free radicals also play key roles in the development of cardiovascular disease. As it turns out, the Mediterranean diet is essentially anti-inflammatory. It is also rich in antioxidants, which, of course, counteract oxidative stress.

Since the initial revelations from the extensive and wide-ranging Seven Countries study, successive generations of scientists have analyzed every conceivable aspect of the traditional Mediterranean diet and lifestyle. Researchers have carefully investigated many of the precise mechanisms by which the diet's various components work together to reduce inflammation, while promoting remarkably good health and statistically significant increases in lifespan.

The benefits appear to derive primarily from two main factors: It is nearly vegetarian, providing ample phytonutrients, natural antioxidants and natural anti-inflammatory compounds, and it is virtually devoid of saturated or trans fats, while also exceptionally low in simple carbohydrates (especially refined sugar). In the mid-1990s the public was reintroduced to the benefits of the diet, after it was popularized by Dr. Walter Willett, a scientist at Harvard University's School of Public Health.

The Mediterranean diet is an overarching term that includes cuisines from a diverse array of countries. It encompasses everything from the succulent and spicy dishes of North African countries like Morocco, Tunisia and Egypt, to the delectable cuisines of Greece, Spain, Italy and

Turkey. Among these countries, Spain and Greece appear to adhere most faithfully to the most beneficial habits of the dietary pattern.

I think it's interesting that fresh herbs are such an important part of Mediterranean cuisine. I suspect that the use of fresh herbs—which Mediterranean cooks take for granted, given that these beloved herbs literally grow like weeds in the agreeable Mediterranean climate—is an important, but often-overlooked component of the diet.

While it's somewhat more challenging for American cooks to keep fresh herbs on hand—and in daily use—it's probably worth the effort. Take fresh oregano, for instance. At last report, more than 450 compounds had been identified in this mint-family herb. More than half of these are natural anti-inflammatory compounds.

Meal Time Is For More Than Just Eating

Another aspect that characterizes the Mediterranean Diet is not just the food or spices used, but the relaxed approach to family centered meals, with an emphasis on enjoying one's food. Smaller portions are also common. Taking time to enjoy your food, and the company of those you share it with, may be just as important as what you eat.

Some of my best memories growing up were those shared at mealtime with my parents and two brothers. One would not eat in a rush to get back to work or school. In fact, in Spain, and many other Mediterranean countries, everything closes down at lunchtime. From 1 p.m. until 4 p.m., the streets are empty, the stores shut down, and everyone is home, having lunch with the family.

I have heard Americans refer to this lunch break as "siesta," which means nap. But the reality is that most people do not take naps on a daily basis, other than the very old and the very young. Adults and children use the extended break to enjoy a leisurely, relaxing meal with family, while relating stories about their morning at school or work. This unhurried time together helps build a good family foundation.

The Mediterranean Diet and Diabetes

In 2010, European scientists published the results of a large, randomized, four-year study on the ability of the Mediterranean diet to prevent diabetes in subjects at high risk of developing cardiovascular disease, compared with a low-fat diet alone. Participants who consumed a Mediterranean diet, which included plenty of extra virgin olive oil or nuts, experienced a 52% drop in the risk of developing diabetes, compared to subjects who ate a low-fat diet alone. None of the subjects lost significant amounts of body weight, or increased their levels of exercise significantly. Nevertheless, people who followed the Mediterranean diet most closely were the least likely to develop diabetes.

Another study looked at the effects of the Mediterranean moderate-fat diet on various markers of inflammation and cardiovascular health, including levels of glycosolated hemoglobin (HbA1C). HbA1C levels are used to estimate patients' long-term blood-sugar control. Higher levels show that blood sugar levels have routinely climbed too high in the preceding weeks or months. Subjects followed the study diet for three months. Various blood components were analyzed, and subjects then switched to their usual diet for three months, followed by more blood tests.

Compared to most subjects' ordinary diets, the Mediterranean diet was associated with a significant decrease in HbA1C levels. Subjects also had higher levels of dietary antioxidants and heart-healthy monounsaturated fats in their bloodstreams while following the Mediterranean diet. The researchers concluded that adherence to the Mediterranean diet improved subjects' blood-sugar control.

According to a recent review of scientific studies on the subject, the majority of existing evidence indicates that adopting the Mediterranean diet may help prevent type 2 diabetes among people who have not yet developed the disease, while also improving glycemic control and reducing cardiovascular disease risks in people who already have diabetes.

Italian researchers noted that two large prospective studies reported substantially lower risks of developing type 2 diabetes among healthy people who most faithfully adhere to the principles of the Mediterranean diet. The decreased risk ranged from a remarkable 83% reduction in one study, to a respectable 35% decrease in the other.

Onions and Apples

If you have had the opportunity to visit Spain, France, Italy or Greece, you will probably recall the scent of fresh onions and garlic, which are used in almost every dish. Apples, which are grown throughout the region, are also a staple ingredient used in many recipes.

One example of a specific element of the Mediterranean diet that works to ensure good health is quercetin. Quercetin is a natural flavonoid that is found in abundance in foods such as onions and apples. According to the results of a study published in the highly respected *British Journal of Nutrition*, quercetin supplementation decreases oxidized LDL-cholesterol and lowers blood pressure in overweight people at risk of developing cardiovascular disease.

LDL-cholesterol is not inherently "bad." Oxidization of LDL-cholesterol is what makes this form of cholesterol problematic. Subjects in the double-blind, placebo-controlled trial received 150 mg of quercetin per day, or an inactive placebo, for six weeks. After a five-week washout period, subjects were switched to the alternate treatment. Subjects' blood pressure and blood lipid profiles were assessed after each phase of the trial.

People with high blood pressure (hypertension) had lower systolic blood pressure while taking quercetin, but not when they consumed the placebo. In a subgroup of adults 25-50 years old, quercetin supplementation yielded an even greater reduction in systolic blood pressure. Quercetin also significantly decreased concentrations of oxidized LDL-cholesterol, which is likely to correlate with a reduced risk of developing atherosclerosis, the root cause of most heart disease.

Our ancestors were doing more than just adding flavor when they ate raw onions and apples, or added them to seasonings and dressings. They were staying healthy.

Red Wine

Of course, the Mediterranean region is also famous for its grapes and wine. Indeed, the world's best wines come from a handful of regions around the world with a Mediterranean-type climate, such as France and Italy, or the Napa and Sonoma Valleys in California, or the wine-growing regions of Australia and Chile. It's not surprising then that wine consumption in moderation is also a characteristic of this lifestyle.

Alcohol consumption in excess is unarguably unhealthy for a variety of obvious reasons, but it's interesting to note that most experts now agree that alcohol consumption in moderation can provide substantial benefits in terms of heart disease prevention. Accordingly, most physicians now recommend that men consume two units of alcohol per day. Women are encouraged to drink one unit of alcohol daily to help preserve cardiovascular health.

A unit of alcohol is roughly defined as one measure (25 milliliters) of hard liquor, one-half pint of regular beer, or one small glass of wine. The recommendations don't apply to recovering alcoholics, or to people who have been diagnosed with certain types of cancer, as alcohol is suspected of encouraging tumor growth in some instances.

Red wine has received plenty of attention for its healthful polyphenol content (primarily resveratrol), but scientists now believe that alcohol itself is responsible for the cardiovascular-protective effects of moderate drinking.

 Secrets to remember:

- Don't rush meals. Eat slowly and enjoy the company.
- Follow the Mediterranean style of limited meat and dairy consumption.
- Indulge in beneficial foods, especially fresh fruits and vegetables.
- Add raw or cooked onions to your meals.
- An apple a day really helps keep the doctor away!
- Drink wine in moderation.

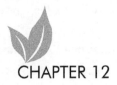

CHAPTER 12

Steps to a Happy, Healthy You

From our own selves our joys must flow...
Nathaniel Cotton

Give yourself permission to be happy. The inner confidence and personal dialogue that we talked about before is one of the secrets to personal happiness. First you have to like yourself. Next you can unconditionally love yourself. I list "like" ahead of love because of its paramount importance.

You may love your mom, your mate, your children or a good friend, yet you may not *like* them. You may wish you could change the way they act, or alter some of the choices they make. I enjoy telling my husband that I like him *and* I love him. I think it's important to like and love anyone you have an important relationship with. The first time I told Mike that I liked him, he gave me a puzzled look. "Yes, I do like you," I continued, and then I explained what I meant. "Many couples that get divorced do it not because they don't love each other anymore, but because they have grown out of their like for each other. Then over time, that dislike transforms into falling out of love."

But what about your inner like for yourself? Many people, men and women alike, have allowed others to dictate how they should feel about themselves, including their appearance. This internal dialogue silently shapes whether or not we like ourselves. And that can affect whether or not we love ourselves. So, what is the secret? How do you steer your internal dialogue towards a healthier, more constructive narrative? The first area I would like to address is weight. Although I am the first one to support the idea of a healthy body weight, over the years I have seen so many people become unhappy and hate their beautiful bodies because they don't fit in a specific dress size or type of clothing.

Although pounds are pounds, there are a number of things to keep in mind. Two women may have the same height and weight, yet look completely different. Why? Because they have different body types and structures.

Women with a larger body frame will typically distribute their pounds differently than those with a smaller one. Also, genetically we are predisposed to have areas with a larger amount of fat cells than others. That's why a dress may not fit the same on two different women, regardless of size.

The point is this: You must like yourself because of your indisputable qualities, your unique abilities, your talent as a mom, a women, a business person. Doing so will allow you to fall in love with you as a person. This is the first step to being happy and having a healthy mind set. Then love yourself. You have something unique, which no one else has. We all do, and the key is to identify that uniqueness and maximize it.

The second step I want you to focus on is the word skinny. I essentially want you to remove it from your vocabulary. Why? Because skinny is not necessarily healthy. Many women you see on TV are so thin that if you saw them in real life without clothing you would not think of them as beautiful, sexy, or healthy in any way. Have you ever hugged someone who's too thin? You give them a little squeeze and it feels like they are going to break. What's attractive about that?

We all like to feel some substance when holding someone. If you don't, you should change your mindset. I am not saying fat or overweight, I am just saying healthy looking, with a little coverage over the bones. We should all work towards that goal and instill these ideals in our children so they won't grow up thinking they are fat when they are not. Eating right to maintain proper weight is important, but *feeling* healthy is probably the single most important thing anyone can do.

So if being skinny is not a healthy goal, what is, you may wonder. The focus must be on vibrant health, which in turn will make you feel happy. Simply aspire to look and feel healthy: neither too fat nor too thin. Just healthy. And teach your children to eat healthful foods, while avoiding empty calories.

Consistently adhering to a good diet has been proven to reduce one's risk of diabetes, heart disease, stroke, high blood pressure, obesity and the metabolic syndrome, among other chronic diseases. Looking good is an admirable goal, but if we want to make a change in our society, we must start at home, with ourselves and our children. Teach your kids that a healthful diet featuring organic produce is also the safest and most satisfying way to avoid accelerated aging and inflammation. The right diet can even reduce your risk of developing cancer, or even Alzheimer's disease at any age.

No single diet is perfect for everyone. Some people are allergic to gluten, a protein found in wheat, wheat products and certain other grains, such as rye and barley. These people will greatly benefit from a gluten-free diet. Celiac disease, a serious condition associated with gluten intolerance, is relatively rare. Only 0.5 to 1% of Americans are estimated to be affected. Other individuals may be lactose intolerant, rendering them unable to tolerate dairy products.

True Nutrition

Katherine Zeratsky, a Mayo Clinic nutritionist, has written that depression and diet may be related. Preliminary research indicates, she notes, that people with a poor diet may be more likely to develop depression. She notes that researchers in Britain investigated the link between depression and diet in more than 3,000 middle-aged office workers. The five year study found that people who ate a junk food diet were more likely to report having symptoms of depression.

Zeratsky also points out that studies have indicated that people who follow a Mediterranean diet are less likely to be diagnosed with Parkinson's and Alzheimer's diseases. Although there are many ways to eat right, I tailored my True Nutrition plan to be not just healthy, but easily doable.

True Nutrition is a Mediterranean Plan with a twist. After years of living here, I have come to realize that although the Mediterranean Diet is a great lifestyle, it is easier to follow if you actually live in the Mediterranean region. Most Americans don't have that opportunity, so my plan features adjustments that still provide True Nutrition, while making it easier for Americans to follow. It is worthwhile to analyze some of the properties of my plan that make it unique. Why reinvent the wheel, when we can just make it fit with a few careful adjustments?

 ## Secrets to remember:

- Unconditionally love yourself.
- Identify your uniqueness and maximize it.
- Skinny is not necessarily healthy.
- Aspire to look and feel healthy: neither too fat nor too thin, just healthy.
- No single diet is perfect for everyone.

CHAPTER 13

Put My Secrets into Practice

Self-trust is the first secret of success.
Ralph Waldo Emerson

My son Micah didn't like eating wild-caught salmon. As a mom who knows the benefits of eating fish, I had to think of a way to get him interested enough to at least try it. I knew if he tried it he would like it, but as you may know, sometimes it's a challenge to get a child to just try something he thinks he doesn't like. I needed a trick; a twist on the ordinary approach that would capture his fancy and overcome his objections.

Using a round metal cookie cutter, I would make little circles of salmon, paint them with melted Boursin® cheese, and top them with a drop of tomato paste. Later, I served them with a little shaped mountain of organic brown basmati rice with broccoli ears, red pepper eye brows, black olive eyes, a mini carrot nose, and an organic mustard smile.

When Micah asked what I had made for dinner, I would not say salmon. I would add a twist and say I made "Cheese Sam". Micah would eat it every time, without complaints. Why? The reality is that he likes salmon, but as a little boy he was reluctant to try new things unless they looked attractive enough to make it worth his while.

Sadly, we don't change all that much as we grow older. If your mother raised you to eat meat and potatoes, that is what you crave and most likely love. It's comforting and familiar. Perhaps you are reluctant to try new foods, even though you might actually like them once you give them a chance and become accustomed to them.

I have close friends, relatives, and acquaintances who simply do not eat many fruits and vegetables. In fact, I have been told, "They go to waste in my refrigerator. My children are more likely to eat a bowl of cereal than a piece of fruit." Someone once even told me, "My son actually loves fruit. It's just that he doesn't like getting it ready." Does this sound familiar? If so, what can you do?

Make It Happen

True Nutrition starts at home, and it falls to mom and dad to make it happen. We simply cannot expect a child to make wise food choices if those habits have not been inculcated since childhood. Even when good habits have been taught, it's easier for a child to reach for the cookie jar than for an apple.

Strong, healthy families make strong healthy nations. The proof is in the pudding. We are becoming a diseased land with alarming childhood obesity rates. Diseases like diabetes and high blood pressure, which once only affected senior citizens, are now common among our children.

The Mayo Clinic says, "High blood pressure in children can develop for the same reasons it does in adults — being overweight, eating a poor diet and not exercising." We worry about our children's future and their education. We look for the best schools, and the most reliable teachers. We want them to be on the football team, to play an instrument, to attend drawing classes, and whatever else we can afford. We do all these things because we love them and we want them to be exposed to new experiences and have a well-rounded education. As parents, we know that whatever they are exposed to as children will have a huge impact on their future. But with so much emphasis on education, we sometimes forget about the basics. Teaching our children about healthful nutrition should be one of those fundamentals. It may be the most important thing they'll ever learn.

We can survive without knowing how to play the piano, or how to pitch a fastball, but one of the first things a baby wants when it enters the world is food. Clearly, the need for food is primal. So why not recognize the importance of this fundamental need, and teach our children to make good choices about food?

Teach Good Habits

Coach your children so they learn the importance of eating a variety of foods; fruits, vegetables, legumes and seeds. Wash most of your fruit and finger-size veggies as soon as you purchase them. Wipe them dry, or let them air dry on the kitchen counter. Hopefully, you can purchase mostly organic products. If you do, be sure to put them in the refrigerator. Since they do not have any preservatives they tend to spoil faster than other produce when left at room temperature.

Once your fruits and vegetables are washed, place them in small containers or bags. You will notice that snacking on healthy produce is much easier for kids when they don't have to go through the trouble of hunting in a drawer inside the fridge.

To make things easier for yourself and your children, make room for a "healthy tray" in your refrigerator. A healthy tray can have things like mini resealable bags with cherries, peeled mandarins, strawberries, nuts, grapes, and carrots. Or try making small 2-ounce containers with smashed bananas mixed with peanut butter, apple sauce and other natural, nutritious foods. Include your little ones in the process. They can help you make the healthy trays, by peeling some fruits, or just handing you nuts to put in bags. Your children will be more likely to reach for these healthy choices if they have participated in the creative process.

A key element is to tell your children that when they are hungry they can pick anything from the healthy tray, but from nowhere else. If you do this regularly, and they know the healthy tray will always contain treats they can eat, they will reach for them. Giving your youngsters the freedom to choose from all those snacks empowers them. It gives them autonomy and helps instill a sense of independence.

These habits also teach your children the difference between healthy and unhealthy foods. Kids must be taught about responsible eating starting at a tender age. You can't expect them to make good choices in the future otherwise. It is our responsibility as parents to do so.

Labels and Serving Sizes

It's also important to interpret nutritional information on food labels and teach your family to do the same. Keep in mind that all the numbers are based on serving size. A label highlighting "only 150 calories per serving" may end up making you eat more. In many cases serving sizes are not realistic. If you are not paying much attention to serving sizes, you may end up eating more than you had planned.

Serving sizes are precise. A cup means a flat cup, not a heaping one. Same for a tablespoon. If you love peanut butter, for example, don't cheat yourself by thinking a heaping tablespoon of peanut butter has only 100 calories. If your tablespoon is heaped high, you are most likely eating 1-½ servings, or closer to two, than the single serving listed on the container. Measure accurately; always remove any excess from the top of your measuring device to ensure you get a realistic serving size.

Serving sizes can be deceiving in other ways, and it takes practice to realize where these deceptions hide. Let's say that one day you want to treat yourself to your favorite, perhaps less-than-ideally-healthful cereal. I have been doing great on my True Nutrition Plan, you tell yourself, so I deserve a small treat. You decide to have just one serving of the yummy, sugary cereal. You read the nutritional facts panel and see that one serving is just 200 calories. So far, so good.

So you pour cereal into your bowl and munch away with relish. You reason that a couple hundred calories for an occasional treat is not so bad. Buoyed by your temporary sugar-high, you glance a bit more closely at the cereal's nutritional information. Two hundred calories is equal to one serving size. And one serving size is three-quarters of a cup. You look at what you still have left, and notice that you just poured a lot more than one sinless serving. You probably had more than two; a whopping 500 calories!

To Count Calories or Not

I don't believe in counting calories, but at the same time I want you to become familiar with how many calories are found in certain foods. That is why I encourage you to measure everything until you become familiar with how many calories are in a specific serving. The idea is to increase your awareness of what you're consuming.

Serving sizes are arbitrary, and calorie content is determined by serving size. How to avoid this common pitfall? It may seem a bit tedious, but once you get in the habit, it becomes second nature. Instead of dispensing foods using tableware spoons or cups, always use measuring implements.

For instance, using a one-quarter cup measure to take cereal out of the box, you will be more likely to fill your bowl with one serving, consisting of just three-quarters of a cup than if you poured the cereal freely into a bowl. I am not exaggerating. Measure everything you eat before eating it. Become familiar with actual "flat on top" serving sizes and be aware of the total calories, the total grams of sugar, fats and carbohydrates and overall nutrients you are eating. You may be surprised to realize how many calories you can save in this manner, just by paying attention.

Something else to keep in mind is that manufacturers aren't concerned about your waistline, your health, or your children's health. To make foods more appealing to consumers, they market serving sizes that are smaller than what most people would actually eat. In reality, they expect that you will eat more than just one serving at a time. That is why some packaged foods will say "one-month supply" or "30 servings," when in reality you will finish them sooner.

Teach your family to measure their foods and read labels. When children learn to interpret labels from childhood, it becomes second nature to be more conscientious about choices. My son who is now eight likes to grocery shop with me. I take the opportunity to make it a fun teaching game. Part of our fun is to make him read the labels and tell me how many total calories, fat calories, sugar grams and so on are in a given item before we'll choose it. He now knows to identify the size of any serving and to tell me whether an item is "healthy," considering the amount of sugar, fat and other ingredients. You can do the same.

Replace Your Plates

Have you ever noticed that in Europe we use smaller lunch and dinner plates, as well as drinking glasses, bowls, coffee cups, and even serving platters? It's true. Dishes themselves tend to be larger in American homes and restaurants than in Europe. You may wonder, what does the size of my plate have to do with anything? The answer is, rather a lot. We eat more when we serve ourselves more, and it's easier to stack an excessive amount of food on a large plate than on a smaller one.

I you struggle with portion control start using smaller plates as soon as possible. With this simple fix, you will reduce your calorie intake. Multiple studies have shown that how much we eat is guided more by sight than by hunger. If food is served on a large plate you may end up eating more, even though you may already be satisfied. This is a problem for many Americans. All those surplus calories can lead to gain weight.

Calories Are NOT All the Same

A study published in June 2012 in the *Journal of the American Medical Association* (JAMA) suggests that the best way to maintain your weight is not by following a low-fat or low-carb diet, but by adhering to a European-style diet resembling the Mediterranean eating lifestyle. This dietary pattern features about 40% carbohydrates, 40% fats, and 20% protein.

I think it's worth noting that the European Type Mediterranean Diet has a famously low glycemic index. The Glycemic Index of foods provides a way to measure how fast blood glucose levels rise after consuming a specific food. For example, glucose itself has a glycemic index of 100. In contrast, whole foods such as beans, most vegetables and some fruits, have a Glycemic Index of less than 55, meaning that they do not raise blood glucose levels quickly. I already talked in Chapter 5: The Bitter Taste of Sugar about the negative side effects of a diet abundant in sugars. The results cannot be ignored: sugar intake is linked to increased triglycerides, increased LDL cholesterol, fatty liver, weight gain, diabetes, heart disease and ultimately death.

True Nutrition Carbohydrates

Whole grains, legumes and *seeds* includes everything from whole wheat and brown rice, to chickpeas and pinto beans, to sesame seeds and quinoa. This category supplies plenty of nutrients, most notably essential amino acids; the building blocks of protein.

Technically a seed, quinoa is a grain-like import from the New World that is one of nature's near-perfect foods. High in fiber and low in fat, this staple of the Incas is a source of complete protein, meaning it supplies all the essential amino acids humans need to thrive; a relative rarity in the plant kingdom. You can use quinoa in the True Nutrition Plan

Wheat is probably native to the Mediterranean region. Flour, made from wheat, is one of the key staple foods that have allowed civilization to blossom. Most of us are familiar with refined, snow-white flour, but whole grains, rather than refined grains, are the more healthful choice. For this reason, when I recommend grains in the True Nutrition Plan, I am referring to whole grains.

Grains like wheat, rye and barley consist of three nutritious layers, including the fiber-rich outer bran layer, the inner core called the endosperm, and a diminutive oil-rich portion called the germ. Refined flour is made by removing the natural bran and germ, but these are highly nutritious, containing much of the grain's fiber and phytonutrients. That's why the True Nutrition Plan features whole, not refined; brown, not white.

If you would like a list of allowed carbohydrates go to my website CocoMarch.com and enter the key words "True Nutrition carbs" to download my free report.

The Fat You Should Use:
Extra Virgin Olive Oil and Olives

This delightful, mildly fruity oil provides the majority of calories from fat in the typical Mediterranean diet, and is included in the True Nutrition Plan. Cuisines vary widely in the region, but olives and extra virgin olive oil are a near-universal feature, if not a hallmark, of the Mediterranean diet as well as my True Nutrition Plan.

I bring my olive oil from a small area near my parents' home in Spain, a county named "El Baix Camp," which belongs to the province of Tarragona. For those of you who are well acquainted with olive oil, as I am, the taste and color vary distinctly from one type of olive to another. In the Baix Camp they grow a variety called Arbequina. The Arbequina olive has a characteristic aroma of mature fruit mixed with fresh herbs. Something remarkable about this type of olive is the slightly sweet flavor, with a hint of almonds, which, incidentally, are also grown in the area.

To make the best Arbequina olive oil, the olives must be handpicked in November while they are still a bit green. Most olives are "cold pressed" at around 27 degrees Celsius (somewhat above room temperature). The oil from the first press is the most desirable. The color is deep green. The greener and more intense the color, the better the quality of the olive oil.

Once olive oil is exposed to heat it loses some of its wonderful qualities. Adding a small amount of raw olive oil to your finished dishes ensures a burst of fresh, complex flavors and antioxidants, while providing just a fraction of the calories you'd get by cooking with it.

When I refer to olive oil, I mean raw olive oil. True Nutrition uses only small amounts of oils for cooking. You can sauté mostly with stocks of chicken or vegetables and very little oil. Cooking with fats is almost always unnecessary, and adds many unwanted calories. Although I suggest the use of oil in some recipes, in most I just add organic chicken or vegetable stock to reduce the need for cooking oils. The final result is that your food will still taste just as good, but with fewer calories.

Health Benefits from Olive Oil

Someone once told me that I glamorize olive oil, and I suppose that's true to some extent. But there are many reasons to do so. It is perhaps not surprising that Spanish and Greek scientists have dominated scientific research into the remarkable health benefits of olive oil, as the diets of people from these countries represent some of the best examples of the traditional Mediterranean diet.

Olive oil is primarily a monounsaturated fat. These are the "good" heart-healthy fats, found almost exclusively in plants. Olive oil is the most representative food of the classic Mediterranean diet, and evidence suggests that it may be the most important. Its constituents are remarkably healthful, as ongoing research continues to prove.

An article published in late 2012, in the *American Journal of Clinical Nutrition (AJCN),* was representative of this research. Spanish scientists evaluated the association between the consumption of olive oil and overall mortality among Spanish people. The scientists found an association between greater olive oil intake and a lower risk of dying. The study concluded that people with the greatest intake of olive oil enjoyed a 26% reduction in the risk of dying from all causes, compared to people with the lowest intake of the oil. While that's impressive enough, the benefits of olive oil consumption were even more remarkable when scientists looked specifically at deaths from cardiovascular disease. Among the biggest consumers of olive oil, there was an astounding 44% lower risk of dying from heart disease compared to non-olive oil eaters.

The study's authors also noted that olive oil consumption appeared to be protective against certain types of cancer, such as breast cancer. Different studies over the years have shown that olive oil possesses numerous phytochemicals, which have antioxidant and anti-inflammatory effects in the body. It is believed that these components may account for the extraordinary healthfulness of this classic Mediterranean staple food.

True Nutrition Protein

My True Nutrition Plan allows for balanced amounts of meat, preferably organic. However, provided one is not lactose intolerant, dairy (particularly in the form of yogurt) can also be a great source of protein. Many people who consider themselves lactose intolerant can tolerate yogurt better than milk. Lactose is a sugar found in milk. It's what provokes unpleasant symptoms among individuals who lack the enzyme, lactase, which is responsible for digesting this milk sugar.

Many people descended from Northern Europeans carry a genetic mutation that allows them to continue digesting lactose throughout their lifetimes. But others, especially people whose ancestors hail from Mediterranean and Asian countries, lose this ability in infancy. They eventually become lactose intolerant. However, yogurt containing live active bacteria has relatively small amounts of lactose. Most people who can't drink milk do just fine with yogurt.

Yogurt is an excellent source of calcium and milk protein, called whey. Whey is a complete protein that may have a stronger effect on satiety (the feeling of fullness) than other sources of protein. This effect on satiety may explain why yogurt can contribute to weight loss/maintenance. In fact, studies have shown that diets featuring regular consumption of yogurt products may promote weight loss and maintenance of a healthy weight, including maintaining more lean muscle mass, while also helping to protect bone health.

Before World War II the diet consumed primarily by rustic people in the Mediterranean region simply did not feature significant amounts of red meat, but it did include regular amounts of dairy. When it was available, meat was often included as a flavoring; a complement to the main dish, rather than as a main course. And that is the way I recommend eating meat, in balanced amounts.

Another reason to make yogurt your primary source for dairy, rather than milk, is that yogurt provides beneficial probiotics. These helpful living organisms help stabilize the microflora in the gut; a shifting and vastly important cast of microbial characters that help us absorb nutrients from our food and protect us from a variety of assaults from harmful bacteria and fungi.

Probiotics

Probiotics in yogurt and other foods help colonize the digestive tract with microorganisms that protect and benefit us. Some studies have shown that regular consumption of yogurt rich in live probiotic cultures is associated with a reduction in digestive disorders, better immune system function, reductions in allergy-related symptoms, and better weight management.

A study in the *International Journal of Cancer* concluded that high yogurt consumption is linked to a significantly lower risk of colorectal cancer, leading investigators to note that yogurt consumption should be considered as a means of preventing the disease. It now seems likely that the high calcium content in dairy also plays a role in dairy's anti-obesity effect, possibly accounting for up to half of the overall beneficial effect of dairy products on weight management.

Choosing the Right Yogurt

I favor Greek yogurt for its high protein content. Ideally, yogurt should always be purchased plain, never sweetened. Flavored yogurts are loaded with unnecessary sugars that provide unwanted empty calories. Yogurts sweetened with artificial sweeteners may not carry the added sugar calories, but they have the negative effects of these poisonous sweeteners, and are simply not worth the taste.

Greek yogurt can be a bit heavy to eat plain, but you can make it taste great by simply adding a little bit of water to make it slightly smoother and a few drops of stevia to make it sweet. If you like more flavor, look for liquid flavors near the spice isle in your local health food store, many of them are even organic. Most stores have a wide variety from fruity ones to vanilla or even chocolate.

I love lemon, and often use organic liquid lemon flavor mixed with my plain Greek yogurt or even add it to my berry fruit smoothies. If you don't want to buy flavoring you can also grate the skin of a lemon or an orange and add it to your yogurt for a pop of flavor.

Add the organic flavoring to taste, plus a few drops of stevia or a package of Truvia and some water, then just stir. You will have a delicious, all natural flavored Greek yogurt with a fraction of the calories (and for less money!)

Sugar Substitutes

Aspartame, Saccharin, and Sucralose (Splenda®) are all artificial sweeteners that should be avoided at all times. Some natural sugar substitutes are Luo han guo, also known as Monk Fruit, Xylitol, Erythritol, and Stevia. Stevia has zero calories and I use it most of the time, either in liquid or powder form.

Truvia®, made by Cargill, is extracted from the plant *Stevia rebaudiana*. It has virtually no aftertaste. In my opinion, it's one of the best tasting stevia products available. Cargill is a privately owned company. We have only limited information about their manufacturing process to make Truvia® from stevia. I am hoping that at some point they will reassure consumers that their manufacturing methods guarantee that Truvia® is natural and safe. However, at this point even though I use

Truvia® occasionally, I don't use it as often as I might, because of the lack of information about their manufacturing processes.

However, if you have to choose between Truvia® and any artificial sweeteners please go with Truvia®, as the source is a plant and not an artificial chemical. Splenda® (Sucralose), aspartame and saccharin are all made chemically and are poisonous to your body. You can also use pure Stevia in liquid or powder form.

All my recommendations in this chapter, and the rest of the book or the free report I provide via my website are based on my own research and experience. I have not been paid or sponsored by any company to promote them or their products. They don't even know they appear in this publication.

I have shared my favorites with you because before choosing them I spent many hours researching and comparing options. In my opinion, my suggestions also take into account the best values when you compare prices. If you have your favorites and you think they should be added to future printings of this book, visit me at CocoMarch.com and send me a message. I will be updating my website with your tips and sharing them to help others. If you'd like to interact with other readers, join my Facebook page.

 ## Secrets to remember:

- True Nutrition starts at home. Teach your children about good nutrition from an early age.
- Serving size matters. Keep an eye on serving sizes, and consider switching to smaller plates to help control portion sizes.
- Extra virgin olive oil is a hallmark of the Mediterranean diet and my True Nutrition Plan. Embrace it in your diet.
- Choose complex carbohydrates from whole grains over simple carbs. Whole foods tend to have a lower glycemic index.
- Yogurt is an excellent source of calcium, complete protein, and probiotics. Choose low- or nonfat.
- Avoid toxic artificial sweeteners. Choose Stevia instead.

PART III

Realistic Supplementation

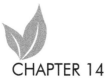

CHAPTER 14

Are Your Vitamins Making You Sick?

It is health that is real...not just gold and silver.
Mohandas K. Gandhi

D iet and lifestyle play a crucial role in health; more so than most people realize. This was eminently clear to me when I began seeing patients here in America. Virtually every complaint, disease or illness I saw could be linked back to patients' poor dietary habits in the previous ten years or so. I worked with patients to reverse any number of illnesses using the transformative power of True Nutrition. I've always tailored individual plans for my patients, but generally my prescription usually included large amounts of fruits and vegetables to be consumed raw, juiced, steamed or in casseroles. I'm a pragmatist, not an idealist, so I always attempted to construct a plan that I knew would fit with an individual patient's schedule. I knew it had to be doable, or they'd simply give up too soon.

As my patients changed the way they behaved—how they shopped, cooked, ate, exercised and thought about taking responsibility for their own health—they began to experience positive improvements, gradually and sustainably. Occasionally, I would prescribe certain dietary supplements, but in most cases I emphasized the role of fresh, organic whole foods in providing everything the body needs to maintain excellent health. I think supplements have their place, and even drugs may be called for in some instances, but for the most part, I believe it's best to get all the beneficial nutrients you need through a healthful diet.

This is in keeping with one of the fundamental tenants of naturopathic medicine: The body is fully capable of healing itself, given the right support. These changes take time, however, and require a level of commitment that is hard to achieve for everyone. Just as lifestyle-related diseases do not develop overnight, natural healing and sustainable well being cannot be achieved instantly.

Depending on the type or severity of a given patient's condition, improvement is generally a long-term project. This approach is admittedly slower than popping a pill. But unlike taking a medication, where symptomatic relief may occur within an hour or less, there are no side effects to the natural approach to wellness, unless you consider a leaner body, more energy and a better outlook on life to be side effects. Unlike the more conventional methods, with my True Nutrition Plan you're truly addressing the underlying *causes* of illness, rather than addressing the *symptoms* alone.

As I said, though, changing your diet overnight can be difficult. Shopping for organic foods is more expensive, and can often seem like a scavenger hunt as you run from store to store trying to find the best, most affordable, most diverse selections of produce and other groceries. Some of my patients were extremely committed and they began reaping the benefits fairly quickly. But others were simply too sick to do the extra work, or even to keep their food down long enough for it to do them any good.

I don't believe in synthetic supplements and that is what the majority of them are, so I wanted to find a food supplement that could assist my patients in their process of achieving health through True Nutrition. I found that at times people just didn't have the time or opportunity to eat fresh fruits and vegetables if they were traveling, or had a busy week and ran out of fresh produce.

This was especially true of cancer patients who were undergoing, or had recently completed, chemotherapy. They simply had no appetite. So, although I believe that organic whole foods prepared fresh and eaten slowly, can and should provide the basis for a lifetime of good nutrition, I also recognized that some people need a more convenient choice to help them on those days when going to the grocery store and buying, washing, chopping and chewing a bunch of fruits and vegetables simply was not an option.

Nutritional supplements can be of great benefit when they supply nutrients that one is not getting through the diet. Personally, my biggest problem with supplements is that most are particularly difficult to absorb. In fact, according to the Physician's Desk Reference, only about 20% of a given pill is actually absorbed into the bloodstream, where it can do any good.

Numerous factors play a role in absorption. Some have to do with the body's inability to break down and catalyze nutrients that have been compressed into pill form. If the goal is to enhance nutrition, it strikes me as wasteful and inefficient to potentially lose as much as eighty percent of what you're paying for every time you swallow it.

The Bottom Line

Call me cynical, but vitamin and supplement companies in general are corporations that manufacture supplements because there is a huge market and lot of potential for growth; we are sicker every day. Just as many centuries ago ancient alchemists were in search of "the elixir of life," we are still searching for the magic potion that will heal our bodies and restore us to health.

When the search turns to supplements, it seems reasonable to seek supplements of natural origin. But are they really all that natural? The more time I spent researching how these so-called "natural supplements" are made, and learning about the companies that make them, the more skeptical I became.

To my surprise, I learned that many of these vitamin manufacturers are quite large. Some have stock holders, while others have partners and investors. No wonder they are able to invest huge amounts of money on marketing, placing ads on digital media and in popular national magazines. The disadvantage to you, the consumer, is that large corporations with fancy advertising campaigns tend to be more focused on dividends than their customers' health. As a result they tout the benefits of their products, when in reality their vitamins may not be all they claim they are.

I spent some time investigating popular supplements sold in drug and grocery stores. I compiled a list of some of the common ingredients found in these supplements by scrutinizing the most trendy vitamins, minerals and nutritional supplements I could find. These are the brands you see advertised on TV, or featured in print ads in slick magazines. These are the names that most Americans trust and buy. People believe they are doing something good for their bodies when they purchase these products. But I wanted to understand what the fine print at the bottom of each label really means.

As I started reading the lists of "other ingredients" on supplement labels I became alarmed to find so many words that I could barely read. But then I also found ingredients that simply don't belong in a healthy supplement intended for consumption. Some of these ingredients include artificial colorants, fillers and other artificial ingredients that are impossible to pronounce unless you're a chemist. Now the question is, are these materials necessary to make a good supplement?

Before judging, I spent a great deal of time doing research. I interviewed manufacturers and learned the procedures involved in developing and manufacturing a supplement. I have to say I learned a lot. I also learned that you don't need to add talc, or corn syrup, or crospovidone, or artificial colorants, to make a healthful supplement. Yet that's what most pills at your local store contain.

I learned that companies use these materials because they are cheap fillers, which makes for inexpensive products. This enables manufacturers to give consumers the impression that they're getting a large bottle of pills for a reasonable price. Consumers feel they are doing something good for their bodies. Taking vitamins is healthy, after all. Isn't it? In reality, many vitamins in pill form can put a lot of unnecessary stress on the liver and kidneys because these organs are forced to flush out all the unnecessary fillers, chemicals and colorants that have been added.

Pill manufacturing requires the use of inactive ingredients called *incipients*, which can help compact and bind the tablets together. Incipients can come from natural sources, but these are more expensive. There is no legitimate need to add artificial colorants, or plastic derivates. Look at the list of ingredients below, then go to your kitchen cupboard or medicine cabinet and read the list of ingredients in fine print on your vitamin supplement.

These ingredients are usually listed under "other ingredients" in very small print. You will be surprised to see how many of these toxic, artificial, manmade chemicals appear on your own label. Again, they're unnecessary. They're only added because they are cheap and provide volume at minimal cost, or add color to make the pill a bit more attractive. Some of the artificial colorings commonly added to these products are derived from petroleum.

I found that supplement brands such as Centrum® or One A Day®, as well as other well recognized and respected names, contain all or some of these unnecessary ingredients. Remember, these compounds are only used as fillers or visual enhancers to make cheap product appear to be more expensive.

Potentially toxic substances in many brands of vitamin pills:

FD&C Yellow No. 6 Aluminum, FD&C Red No. 40 Aluminum Lake, FD&C Blue #2 Lake, corn syrup, talc, sucrose, crospovidone, hypromellose, sodium aluminosilicate, polyethylene glycol, polyvinyl alcohol, stannous chloride, cellulose, croscarmellose sodium, titanium dioxide, dicalcium phosphate, hydrogenated soybean oil, magnesium stearate, corn starch.

My research left me a little disheartened. How could I in good conscience suggest that anyone purchase products that may contain harmful chemicals? Russell Blaylock, MD, CCN (Certified Clinical Nutritionist) is a retired neurosurgeon and author who also happens to be an expert in nutrition and food additives. Regarding food colorings, Dr. Blaylock says the following food colorings should be avoided. The reason? Many are associated with brain injury and behavioral problems in children, while some cause cancer in laboratory animals. They include: FD and C Blue No. 1, FD and C Green Nos. 2 and 3, Red dye No. 2, FD and C Yellow No. 6, FD and C Yellow No. 5

(Tartrazine), as well as all aluminum lakes; FD and C Yellow, No. 5 Aluminum Lake, FD and C No. 3 Aluminum Lake and FD and C Yellow No. 6 Aluminum Lake.

So if these colorants are associated with cancer and other behavioral issues, does it make sense to consume them in your vitamin supplement? Dr. Josh Axe, is a wellness expert and author of The Real Food Diet Cookbook. In an article titled "4 Dangerous (and Common) Vitamin Fillers You Must Avoid," Dr. Axe notes that titanium oxide is a naturally occurring oxide of the element titanium. As you can see from the previous list, it is used as a pigment in many vitamins. But emerging research suggests that it may interfere with immune system function, says Dr. Axe. He voices my own confusion over this issue, asking why anyone would take a supplement to improve their health if it contains fillers such as these that may negatively impact health. It just doesn't make sense. I could go on, but suffice it to say that these unnecessary fillers should not be there, they don't *need* to be there, and you should not purchase supplements that contain them.

Wrapping my head around all this information about pills was rather overwhelming; it took me a while to realize that I should avoid telling patients to purchase supplements in a pill form. Since 80% of most pills is not absorbed, and many of these supplements are packed with dangerous colorants and fillers, it's hard to justify spending money on such products.

Liquid Supplements

Reasoning that liquids are likely to be better absorbed, I delved into this subject with considerable optimism. I thought it would be wonderful to find a supplement that could help people get the natural nutrients available in fruits and vegetables. I knew I could recommend such a product for my patients to use on days when they had to travel, or were too busy to consume fresh produce.

I learned that liquids are absorbed quickly; about ninety-eight percent of all liquids are absorbed within a few minutes of consumption. This fact was crucial to the next step in my career, which I'll describe in greater detail shortly. Although I had high hopes for liquid supplements initially, as I got deeper into my research on the subject, I became disenchanted with the idea. Three factors influenced my opinion: pasteurization, sugar and sodium benzoate.

Pasteurization: In 1800, when many people were dying from infectious diseases, French chemist and researcher Louis Pasteur showed that the growth of microorganisms was to blame for the spoilage of beverages such as milk and wine. He created a process for killing most undesirable bacteria and fungi. It involves bringing the liquid to a specific temperature for a precise length of time, followed by immediate cooling. Although it does not kill all bacteria, the process greatly reduces spoilage, extending the shelf life of various liquids. It also reduces the risk of food-borne illnesses. Known as pasteurization, the process quickly gained acceptance. It is now practiced routinely throughout the world.

This tale is one of the better known science success stories of the past few centuries. Pasteur's process has undoubtedly helped save countless lives over the years. But there is a little-known downside to pasteurization. While it kills potentially harmful pathogens (disease-causing microbes) it also destroys some beneficial enzymes and friendly, probiotic microbes that occur naturally in food. Digestive enzymes and beneficial phytonutrients that are sensitive to high temperatures are irretrievably lost. This troubled me, as I wanted to include as many naturally occurring enzymes and intact nutrients as possible in any formula I recommended for my patients. I considered it critical, in fact, that they receive these unadulterated natural substances.

I had learned that modern liquid supplements are manufactured using pasteurization to prevent fermentation and reduce bacterial overgrowth. While I understand the logic of incorporating pasteurization into the manufacturing process for these supplements, I also knew it rendered them undesirable for my purposes. Patients recovering from cancer need large amounts of micronutrients. If they are not going to get them from food, due to cancer-related poor appetite, I knew I needed to offer them something that came as close to approximating the benefits of fresh, real fruits and vegetables as possible.

Sodium Benzoate: I also learned that most liquid supplements contain a chemical preservative called sodium benzoate. The research is somewhat unclear, but it appears that when sodium benzoate is in the presence of ascorbic acid (vitamin C), sodium and potassium benzoate may form benzene, a known carcinogen. Additional research in the area of hyperactivity and its relationship to sodium benzoate uncovered a potential link to hyperactivity among children when sodium benzoate occurs alongside additive colorants.

Sugar: I have yet to find a liquid supplement that contains no sugar (or artificial sweeteners), which is also palatable to most people's taste buds. Sugar is probably one of the worst things anyone with cancer can eat, so I certainly didn't want to recommend it to my patients. I found that many liquid supplements have as much as 20 grams of added sugar per serving, some even more. These are not naturally occurring sugars from fruit, but sugars mixed with everything else to cover up the unpleasant taste of the ingredients.

I was back to square one. I was convinced that I couldn't recommend liquid supplements. There are simply too many red flags. I needed to find an alternative for my patients, who clearly needed the benefits of fruits and vegetables in their diet, and were evidently not getting as many of these beneficial nutrients as they should.

Powders

Since pills and liquids were not an option I decided to examine the possibility of using powders for my patients' needs. Powders would not need to be pasteurized, nor would there be a need to add preservatives, as the hydrolyzation process preserves most nutrients.

For any food or nutrient to be of use, it must be absorbed into the bloodstream. Many potentially beneficial nutritional supplements— including vitamins, minerals and antioxidants—are poorly absorbed, so I paid special attention to the *bioabsorption* profiles of the available fruit and vegetable powders that I might be able to recommend to my patients.

At the time there were a few "health food" powdered supplement products on the market, and I was pleased to discover products that were free of fillers, colorants or added sugars. Here was something that might work for my patients, I figured. I was elated.

I explained the benefits of powders over pills or liquids to all my patients and I recommended these so-called "Green Powder Drinks". But they didn't go over well. I sampled a few and quickly discovered that, while the products commercially available at the time may have supplied some useful phytonutrients, they tended to taste simply awful, not to mention looking (and sometimes smelling) like swamp water.

Needless to say, no one likes to drink something nasty, but when you are already nauseated by chemotherapy drugs the last thing you want is to choke down algae-tinted swamp water. I was discouraged. I wanted to mentor my patients in their quest for health, but had come up against this obstacle. They needed a source of easily-prepared, naturally high-antioxidant fruit and vegetable extracts, but the available sources were dismal. Again I had come up against a wall. I was back to square one. Or maybe not.

 Secrets to remember:

- Many commercially available vitamins and dietary supplements feature preservatives, additives, fillers and other "excipients" of questionable value.
- Some common supplements include synthetic dyes made from petroleum products. These dyes have been implicated in hyperactive behavior and other ill effects among some children.
- Pasteurization may alter the nutritional profile of a supplement, killing off potentially beneficial probiotics, for example.

CHAPTER 15

The Genesis of a Revelation

No problems, only solutions.
John Lennon

Diligence: Doing your best to make your best better.
Cocó March

When we are between a rock and a hard place, it may appear that the situation only offers unacceptable solutions. But I don't give up that easily.

I found it puzzling that no one made a powdered supplement drink that was palatable when prepared by mixing with water, rather than high-sugar juices. Most people needed to add sweet juice to help mask the awful taste and smell of the all-natural powder products I found on the market.

One cup of juice contains an average of 120 calories, sometimes even more. That translates to as many as 25 grams of sugar in just one single 8-fluid ounce cup. Remember the research by Dr. Robert Lustig, professor of clinical pediatrics at U.C. San Francisco? Lustig recommends that women consume only 100 calories of added sugar daily. He says men should consume no more than 150 added sugar calories. Practically speaking, this means men and women should consume no more than 25 and 37.5 grams of added sugar per day, respectively. Logically, I could not recommend a powder that needed to be mixed with juice.

I am a solution oriented person. I realized that I had to solve this problem for the benefit of my patients. Somewhat desperate, I began researching the subject, learning everything I could about how to go about making a superb, convenient supplemental food product that actually tastes *good*, rather than just *good for you*. But my powdered True Nutrition blend would need to be free of sugar or chemicals. I spent more than a year just researching ingredients and refreshing my knowledge of plant chemistry. I had never planned to get into the nutritional supplement arena, but circumstances had forced my hand. I needed a nutritional supplement I could offer to my patients in full confidence.

Eventually, I partnered with a laboratory that allowed me to experiment. Like a master perfumer creating an intoxicating new scent, I scrutinized every requisite component. I evaluated various combinations of nutrients not only for their high antioxidant values, but also for their flavors and sensual appeal. Since I insisted on enhancing flavor with natural and organic ingredients, rather than any artificial chemicals, the process was painstaking; a true labor of love.

True Nutrition

When creating my blend I put all my energy and effort into not just creating another version of the typical powered greens nutritional supplement, but into reinventing it altogether. I focused on making something good better. As I mentioned, other "greens" powders were already on the market. They had good ingredients, but what they didn't have was good taste or texture. They were thick, smelly and just plain nasty tasting. I knew that going with powder was the solution, since it provides for quick absorption with minimal processing. Finally the end of my quest was in sight. I could finally offer a truly healthful supplement without unwanted fillers or unnatural additives.

Naming a product is often one of the last steps involved in its creation, but I'd like to address the name of my nutritional supplements first. Various products already existed that incorporated the concept of fresh greens in their name. I kept this reference to capitalize on the fact that my flagship product would supply the kind of naturally healthful nutrition available in the fresh produce aisle, minus the hassle of buying, cleaning, storing and preparing these whole foods. My products supply natural enzymes, trace minerals, probiotics, fiber, phytonutrients, and antioxidants equivalent to 20 servings of fruits and vegetables.

I named my brand Dr. Coco's Delicious Greens. Let me tell you why. I added "delicious" to emphasize the fact that my products are not only palatable, but truly flavorful and, well, delicious. The term "greens" reflects the fact that my blends contain dozens of different greens, which have been dried at low temperature and blended together. Most of my formulas are high ORAC; on average 8000 units per serving. ORAC (*Oxygen Radical Absorbance Capacity*) is a standardized method used to quantify the antioxidant capacity of a given substance.

Without a table of ORAC values for comparison, the number 8,000 may mean relatively little to you. To put this number in perspective, it may be helpful to consider the average ORAC values of some common foods. For instance, one small apple may yield 250 ORAC units, while one serving of watermelon contains approximately 150 units. Each scoop of Delicious Greens contains over 8,000 ORAC units. That's equivalent to the antioxidants found in as many as 20 servings of fruits and vegetables.

Although the Food and Drug Administration does not officially recognize the applicability of ORAC values in foods once they enter the body (beyond those supplied by vitamins A, C, and E), these phytonutrient antioxidants are believed to help fight free radicals. As we've seen, research suggests that free radicals are the culprits behind many diseases, and possibly even aging.

How Dangerous Are Free Radicals?

In Chapter 8, I compared electrons to shoes. Remember the analogy, in which your feet are molecules and your two shoes are electrons? If you were missing one shoe you would be considered "reactive;" you would be a free radical, desperately seeking to steal someone else's shoe to wear, so you could regain your own balance. But in so doing, you would make that person a free radical. Your only solution would be to find a shoe donor, someone with a generous supply of extra shoes. This donor could freely give you the shoe you needed, without becoming another free radical in the process. Having these generous donors circulating stops the destructive cycle of shoe stealing and creation of yet more free radicals.

In this analogy, people with missing shoes are free radicals, while generous shoe donors are antioxidants. The more antioxidants you have in your body the greater the power to neutralize free radicals, and the less damage they're likely to do. This process of molecules losing electrons and causing damage to other molecules to get those missing electrons back happens millions of times each day in our bodies. That is why, if the cycles are not stabilized, they create a vicious sequence of stealing electrons from healthy molecules, and turning those molecules into new free radicals, which in turn have to steal more electrons from other molecules.

As you can imagine, if there were millions of people stealing each other's shoes every minute of every day, you'd start watching your step mighty carefully. And that is how closely we need to watch our health and increase our antioxidant consumption. This is best achieved by eating plenty of fruits and vegetables, or by supplementing with Dr. Cocó Delicious Greens when you don't have the opportunity to eat enough fruits and vegetables.

Oxidative stress is thought to foster both accelerated aging and degenerative diseases. High-fat/high-calorie meals result in significant oxidative stress, but even digesting the leanest of protein can yield a net oxidative effect in the body, at least temporarily. Dietary antioxidants are believed to act like antidotes to oxidative stress by mopping up free radicals.

Delicious Greens Is Not a Multivitamin

My signature *Delicious Greens* nutritional supplement powder provides a wide range of organic foods in a single, easy-to-consume package. It's very expensive to make, but I refuse to cut corners. I've divided the various components into groups, according to their functions. I'll discuss some select ingredients, providing explanations of their benefits, including relevant scientific research that supports these claims.

My formulas are created to supply you with protective antioxidants, although they contain naturally occurring vitamins and minerals, obtained from their ingredients: raw plant extracts, fruits, vegetables, fibers and herbs. Although rich in all types of phytonutrients, Delicious Greens is not a multivitamin. It is not intended to replace your daily multivitamin supplement.

I have been asked why Delicious Greens cannot replace a multivitamin. Food is divided into food groups (*macronutrients*) like proteins, fats and carbohydrates. Even though they all have different roles in the body, they all are equally important. In fact, we cannot live without any of them. In the same manner, *micronutrients* are also divided into groups. Of these groups, the main ones are vitamins, minerals and antioxidants. Delicious Greens furnishes your body with plenty of protective antioxidants, which help energize your body while aiding in cellular repair. But Delicious Greens lacks sufficient vitamins and minerals to be called a multivitamin.

Color and Sweetness

The color of the powders, as well as the sweetness, is a result of the different plants I use. None of my powder mixes contain added sugar. Rather, I use a plant called Stevia to give it a hint of sweetness. I also have Stevia-free blends, which have a naturally fruity taste.

The ingredients in my products provide characteristics such as sweetness and color. These vary by season, however, depending on when the ingredients are harvested. Sometimes fruits and vegetables are more ripe, other times less so. So the coloring and sweetness varies slightly from batch to batch.

Always Fresh

You can find my Delicious Greens formulas in most health food stores and malls around the country. However, you will be guaranteed to get the freshest Delicious Greens when ordering directly from my website, www.CocoMarch.com.

Unlike most product makers, I manufacture our Delicious Greens blends once a month, rather than a couple of times per year, even though making fewer batches less often would be more cost effective. I do this because I want my products to be as fresh as possible. My products have a three-year shelf life, but I highly recommend that you buy them as fresh as you can. Doing so will guarantee the highest spectrum of nutrients should you end up storing the products for a while after purchasing.

My goal is to help you achieve better health, not to become a large corporation that's only concerned about the bottom line. I really want you to feel the difference after using Delicious Greens. That is why I will only provide you with super fresh Delicious Greens that have been manufactured a few days to no more than a few weeks before you order from my website.

Dr. Cocó Organic Greens

Delicious Greens is 100% natural. It is made with non-GMO ingredients and mostly Certified Organic Fruits and Vegetables. However, it contains a number of ingredients and concentrated extracts such as Milk Thistle, Quercetin, and Red Wine or Grape Seed extract, which do not exist in organic form. When creating the formula I chose to use those materials for their natural detoxification benefits. But I had to sacrifice the "organic" labeling, because the final formula was not 95% organic.

However, I also created Dr. Cocó Organics, which is made with only Certified Organic Ingredients; you can chose which formula fits your circumstances. Both formulas contain Certified Organic fruits and vegetables, but Delicious Greens contains some non-organic ingredients, while Dr. Coco's Organic only features organic ingredients.

Delicious Greens and Dr. Cocó Organic Greens are both made from a collection of raw organic plant foods with a variety of wholesome benefits. Powder extracts from vegetables like carrot, broccoli, cauliflower, and parsley give the blends essence and nutrition. Next, I'll share with you some of the potential health benefits of a few of these ingredients, so you'll see why I carefully selected them to be included in my formulas.

Disclaimer

The benefits I list below are those for the individual ingredients as plants, not of my formulas. Delicious Greens and Dr. Coco Organic Greens, as well as all my other powder mixes, are supplements. They are not intended to cure or treat diseases, or to replace the advice of your doctor. I wrote this book for informational purposes only. As I told you before, information is power. What you do with that power is up to you.

When I state that a specific plant has been shown to have anti-cancer properties, I am not making a claim about my product. I am simply sharing with you some of the findings published by independent researchers from universities and other institutions around the world. These scientists have often spent years investigating the properties of specific phytonutrients. Many of these nutrients appear to possess beneficial properties, and that's why you should make sure you eat plenty of them daily.

Cruciferous Vegetables

Broccoli, cauliflower and parsley are all members of the Brassica family of plants. Also known as cruciferous vegetables, these remarkable plants are the source of a number of highly beneficial compounds, which have been linked to potent anti-cancer, antioxidant and anti-atherogenic (atherosclerosis-preventing) activities in laboratory and animal studies.

Beneficial constituents in cruciferous vegetables include compounds called glucosinolates. These are metabolized in the body into other beneficial compounds, including sulforaphane, indole-3-carbinol (I3C) and diindolylmethane (DIM). All are biologically active chemicals that have been credited for providing some of the amazingly healthful benefits of eating broccoli and related vegetables.

Some of these compounds are presently undergoing intense scientific scrutiny, due to their important effects in the body. The National Cancer Institute, for example, is conducting clinical trials investigating the therapeutic effects of DIM against various forms of cancer. Evidence strongly suggests that these natural dietary compounds work in a variety of ways—attacking cancer from a number of angles, as it were—to prevent cancer.

Even among people who have already developed cancer, these compounds can help. They've been shown to improve the effectiveness of chemotherapy drugs during cancer treatment. Besides these natural anti-cancer compounds, cruciferous vegetables are rich sources of various vitamins (E, C and K), minerals (iron, zinc and selenium) and polyphenols, such as quercetin. While the unique contributions of glucosinolates and sulforaphanes in cruciferous vegetables tend to get all the attention, it would be a mistake to underestimate the potential contributions of these other constituents to overall health.

Immune System Support

Delicious Greens and Dr. Cocó Organics also contain custom blends of natural plant extracts and whole, freeze-dried powders chosen for their ability to support immune system function. These include SDG (Secoisolariciresinal Diglucoside) lignans, Red beet root powder, Aloe Vera leaf powder, Cinnamon powder, Mangosteen fruit powder, Açai berry powder, Gogi juice powder, Concord grape powder, Acerola cherry powder, Milk Thistle seed extract (also known as Silymarin), Pomegranate, Turmeric rhizome extract (curcuminoids) Atlantic kelp powder, decaffeinated green tea extract (with active polyphenols), Quercetin a natural bioflavonoid with excellent allergy benefits and Polygonum cuspidatum (supplying Trans-resveratrol found in grapes)

Some of these ingredients may be familiar to you, while others may sound like Greek. SDG lignans, for example, probably sounds like some sort of indigestible filler chemical, but it's not. Actually, it's one of the bioactive components of beneficial plant foods, like flax seed, that are credited with a number of health benefits, including anti-cancer activity. In fact, I assure you, all of the ingredients in my dietary supplement formulas are there for a reason, and all come directly from nature. Next, I'll describe the specific benefits of a number of the ingredients I've included in my various *Delicious* products.

Açai

You've probably heard some mention in the media, in recent years, of açaí (ah-sigh-ee) berry. This rainforest fruit received a massive amount of press a few years back, seemingly taking the "superfoods" headlines by storm. And with good reason. Açaí is a tart berry that's organically grown and sustainably harvested from palm trees in the Amazon rainforest, and it is packed with antioxidants and other nutrients.

A recent animal study published in the journal *Nutrition* looked at the effects of adding açaí powder to the diets of rats that scientists use as a model for the effects of high blood cholesterol levels in humans. After six weeks, rats that received the açaí powder in their feed had higher levels of antioxidants in their bodies, and lower cholesterol levels, than control rats, which ate a similar diet, minus the açaí supplement.

Another recent study, conducted on human subjects, and reported in the *Journal of Medicinal Foods*, looked at the effects of drinking a fruit/berry drink fortified with açaí pulp on pain and range of motion among people with age-related arthritis. After three months of daily consumption, subjects experienced significant increases in their antioxidant levels, as well as improvements in pain, range of motion and other measures of quality of life.

Cinnamon

Cinnamon provides a hint of flavor to my blend, to be sure, but its benefits go beyond mere flavoring. Cinnamon is a relatively unheralded—one might even say underestimated—superfood. Of course, it's been popular for centuries. Prized for its unique flavor and heady scent, cinnamon is surely among the most beloved of spices. Its scent can evoke fond memories of crisp fall afternoons spent sipping cider, and joyous family gatherings accented with cinnamon-laced baked goods. There may be nothing more American than apple pie, but what would that pie taste like without the right hint of cinnamon?

Clearly we love the taste and scent of this ancient spice, but it might come as a surprise to you that cinnamon has health benefits, too. In fact, scientists have discovered that cinnamon has all kinds of beneficial properties, ranging from decreasing inflammation, to suppressing the growth of microorganisms like bacteria and viruses, to improving blood insulin levels, fighting tumor growth, and lowering cholesterol levels.

According to a comprehensive meta-analysis of controlled trials published in late 2011, cinnamon improves fasting blood glucose levels among pre-diabetic and diabetic patients. Investigators examined data collected during eight clinical trials, and concluded that cinnamon and/or cinnamon extract intake yields a statistically significant decrease in fasting blood glucose levels. Fasting blood glucose is a test used to determine the extent by which a person's blood sugar levels drop after 12 hours of fasting.

Milk Thistle Seed Extract

Milk thistle seed extract sounds unappetizing, I'll admit, but it's health-promoting potential is nothing short of amazing. Would you believe this plant has been used to support liver function for 2,000 years? It's true. For centuries, folk healers knew that this plant offered the only hope of survival for unfortunate patients who unwittingly consumed Death Cap (*Amanita* species) mushrooms.

Death Caps are loaded with deadly toxins that overwhelm the liver's ability to neutralize them. Folk healers may not have known exactly how it worked, but we now understand that natural compounds in milk thistle can dramatically boost the liver's ability to incapacitate poisons. Thus were they able, with quick action and a pinch of luck, to tip the balance between certain death and survival.

The extract of this common plant provides a substance called silymarin, which is credited with a variety of beneficial activities. Silymarin itself is a mixture of natural plant compounds called flavonoids; all three are believed to boost the natural antioxidant capability of the liver.

This is important, because the liver plays a crucial role in the body, detoxifying a broad range of potentially harmful chemicals, allowing them to be eliminated before they can cause harm. This includes everything from poisonous mushrooms, to pesticide and herbicide residues in food, to artificial preservatives, to alcohol, medications, and even second-hand toxins from cigarette smoke.

Laboratory and animal studies suggest that silymarin also helps prevent cancer. It may even help protect brain cells from additional damage following stroke. Other studies have suggested that it may help protect against Alzheimer's disease.

Turmeric Root Powder

Since ancient times, people have cultivated, harvested and valued the root of a plant known as *Curcuma longa*. You are perhaps most familiar with the common name of the ground dried rhizome, turmeric. Turmeric is a canary-yellow, earthy-tasting spice familiar to cooks as the basis of any curry seasoning blend.

Although it is perhaps one of the lesser known spices among American cooks, turmeric has taken center stage in the cuisines of many

Asian cultures, where it is consumed virtually every day in one form or another. Aside from curry dishes, Americans are perhaps most familiar with turmeric as the ingredient that puts the sunny yellow color in prepared mustards.

To some extent, it's a shame that we haven't embraced this particular superfood more enthusiastically in this country. Turmeric is the source of a family of compounds called curcuminoids, and these amazing chemicals, like many natural pigments, are highly beneficial. Turmeric's very name hints at its benefits. Turmeric is a corruption of the original name in Latin; *terre merite*, which roughly translates as "worthy earth."

The ancients revered turmeric for its health-promoting and healing properties, and their faith was well placed. Modern scientists across the planet are busily investigating the myriad properties of this humble root. What they've discovered is nothing short of amazing.

Curcumin (a general term for the various active compounds in turmeric) has properties that include: anti-inflammatory, antioxidant, antimicrobial, antiviral and anticancer activities. Curcumin not only reduces inflammation, a process believed to underlie many degenerative diseases, from heart disease to diabetes and cancer, but it also reduces oxidative stress and impedes the development of cancer on multiple levels. This latter property is perhaps of most interest to scientists worldwide.

In laboratories at universities and private research facilities, scientists are actively investigating the specific mechanisms of action involved in curcumin's ability to thwart the development of cancer. These mechanisms appear to be numerous. Because it is an ancient spice with a long history of common use, entrepreneurs cannot patent curcumin for marketing as an anticancer drug. But some companies are attempting to modify certain constituents of curcumin in an effort to do just that.

One of the drawbacks of curcumin as a medicinal herb is its relatively low bioavailability. Bioavailability refers to the degree to which a given plant chemical is absorbed into the bloodstream, and allowed to circulate, after consumption. When you use the spice in cooking, you undoubtedly get some small benefit, but bioavailability is relatively poor. For this reason, I have included a dried concentrate made from the natural rhizome, for improved bioavailability.

Curcumin is exceptionally safe and even in high doses it is very well tolerated. I could go into great detail regarding the many remarkable way in which curcumin works to defend against cancer, from start to finish, and how it can even help in the treatment of cancer after it's established, but I will resist the impulse to provide what could easily become too much information!

Suffice it to say that this is one of the most important superfoods known to man. And that's not hyperbole. Even a cursory review of the medical literature reveals literally thousands of articles and studies that have been written about curcumin in the past few years alone. Scientists are clearly excited about the multifaceted benefits of this ancient spice. And that's why I included it in my formulations. I wanted to make it easy for everyone to take advantage of nature's natural healing bounty.

Green Tea

Water is the most widely consumed beverage on earth. Tea comes in a close second. Billions of people have enjoyed green tea for millennia; it's been used as a health tonic for nearly as long. Green tea consists of the dried green, unfermented leaves of the *Camellia sinensis* shrub, steeped in hot water.

Black tea, which is made from the fermented leaves of *Camellia sinensis*, has somewhat lower concentrations of some of the most healthful compounds found in green or white teas. White tea is made from the delicate new leaf buds of the plant. Beneficial compounds may be even more concentrated in white tea.

Many brews have been called "tea" over the years, but the drink made from *Camellia sinensis* leaves and buds is true tea. This important plant, which is native to China, has been lovingly cultivated for thousands of years. People enjoy the delicate, almost floral fragrance and flavor of green tea, but they also appreciate its reputation as a refreshing beverage that is both invigorating and calming.

This may seem paradoxical, as these qualities appear to be mutually exclusive, but tea's reputation is well deserved. Tea contains caffeine, which is well known for its stimulant properties. But tea also contains a unique amino acid, called theanine, which works to help people relax and feel calm, yet focused. This unique combination of phytochemicals accounts for tea's calming, yet invigorating properties.

But tea's benefits don't stop there. In the past few decades scientists the world over have investigated tea's antioxidant compounds, called flavins, with what can only be described as great enthusiasm. Scientists are excited about these chemicals for a good reason. One in particular, a *catechin* compound called epigallocatechin gallate (EGCG), is a potent antioxidant polyphenol that probably accounts for many of green tea's most remarkable health benefits. These include anticancer activity, and possible anti-diabetes and obesity-fighting effects. The average cup of green tea contains about 235 mg of health-promoting catechins.

In recent years, scientists have amassed mounting evidence to support the hypothesis that green tea helps fight obesity and diabetes. Australian scientists published a comprehensive statistical analysis combining data from a wide range of disparate studies in the *Archives of Internal Medicine, in 2009.* The study examined the diabetes-fighting effects of coffee and tea consumption, and it included data from nearly 300,000 individuals. The study's authors concluded that drinking four cups of decaffeinated tea every day is linked to a 20% reduction in the risk of developing diabetes. Statistically speaking, every cup of tea or coffee consumed was associated with a 7% reduction in relative risk.

In another article, published in the *Journal of the American College of Nutrition,* German researchers reported that obese men who consumed EGCG experienced higher rates of fat burning (thermogenesis) than control subjects who didn't get EGCG. Although it was a small pilot study, with a limited number of participants, it was also a well-controlled study, meaning its design was randomized, double-blind, and placebo-controlled.

This type of study design is regarded as the gold standard among scientists. The researchers concluded that EGCG in green tea probably contributes to tea's reported anti-obesity effects, due to its influences on fat oxidation and thermogenesis.

Chinese researchers reported that green tea reduces DNA damage caused by free radicals, not only in cultured human white blood cells growing in the laboratory, but in live human subjects. The researchers reported a decrease in cellular DNA damage of about 20% due to green tea. DNA damage is thought to play a role in the development of cancer, so the results hint at green tea's cancer-fighting properties.

Obesity is linked to a greater incidence of both diabetes and cardiovascular disease, and both of these conditions are known to involve inflammation. Recognizing this, scientists at the University of California, Davis, showed that EGCG directly reduces inflammation by promoting the production of regulatory T cells.

These immune system cells are important regulators of inflammation, helping put the brakes on runaway inflammation, in a manner of speaking. In obese people these cells are somewhat suppressed. By helping boost their numbers, EGCG exerts a natural anti-inflammatory effect.

Scientists are eager to see data from large controlled human trials. But studies on animals that are commonly used as models of human diabetes clearly show that green tea and its extracts have potent anti-diabetic effects. In one such study, scientists reported that eight weeks of supplementation with EGCG lowered blood sugar, reduced oxidative stress and normalized serum lipids in animals that received EGCG, compared to control animals that did not consume the green tea chemical. In another study, researchers noted that rats fed a high-fructose diet laced with green tea extract did not develop insulin resistance, while rats fed a similar diet without green tea did develop insulin resistance.

Trans-resveratrol

Resveratrol (technically; *trans-resveratrol*) is a fascinating chemical made by certain plants to protect them from a variety of threats. In grapes, for instance, resveratrol evidently guards against potential damage from too much ultraviolet radiation. In effect, it acts as a natural sunscreen. But it also helps grapevines fight off one of the chief threats to their health: fungal infections.

Resveratrol received a huge amount of attention in the media a few years ago, after scientists revealed that it dramatically extends the lifespans of certain lower animals when added to the diet. Of course, extending the lifespan of a flatworm by 50% is one thing, while significantly extending human lifespan is another. But ongoing research suggests that resveratrol does, in fact, exert some remarkably beneficial effects on humans.

Hundreds of studies have examined resveratrol's effects and mechanisms of action in creatures ranging from fungi to human cells. These ongoing investigations are gradually shedding light on the remarkable potential benefits of this phytochemical.

For example, mounting evidence already indicates that this multifunctional plant polyphenol compound helps to protect the cardiovascular system. It's also been shown to improve insulin sensitivity. Resveratrol also improves insulin production and protects against, or at least delays, the development of type 2 diabetes. This is of particular importance given that the number of people with pre-diabetes and type 2 diabetes continues to rise inexorably in this country, and throughout the developed world.

I think it's especially interesting to note that grapevines grown organically, without the use of artificial pesticides, fungicides or herbicides, invariably produce higher concentrations of resveratrol than vines treated with these chemicals. This is yet another example of the ways in which organic produce may be superior to produce raised using modern farming methods, which rely on artificial chemicals to boost yield. Not only are these grapes free of potentially troublesome chemicals, but they are naturally higher in the plant's own chemical, which we now know is highly beneficial not only to the plant itself, but to humans as well.

Studies on both animals and humans have shown that resveratrol helps reverse atherosclerosis, the inflammatory condition underlying most heart disease. Understandably, we all fear cancer. But keep in mind that heart disease is still the *number one* killer in America. Cancer of all types combined still comes in second as a cause of death.

That's not to say that resveratrol can't help protect against cancer, though. Although preliminary, laboratory studies clearly show that resveratrol targets cellular processes involved in the regulation of growth, controlled cell death (apoptosis), cellular differentiation and energy production. These are all processes that play a role in the control—or development—of cancer. Resveratrol appears to help normalize these functions, and this probably means that it also helps protect against cancer.

Resveratrol is found in grapes and grape products, which probably accounts for at least some of the heart-healthy benefits of drinking wine in moderation. It also occurs in a few other plants, such as peanuts and an herb called Japanese knotweed (*Polygonum cuspidatum*), which is the source of the trans-resveratrol that I include in my products.

I find it interesting that resveratrol simulates the effects of calorie restriction to a great degree. In creatures ranging all the way from the simplest fungi to highly intelligent primates, calorie restriction improves a broad range of key health indicators, from lipid levels to blood sugar levels, to antioxidant balance and even lifespan. Scientists have discovered that resveratrol is a "sirtuin activator."

Sirtuin activators are chemicals that trigger the production of proteins called sirtuins. Sirtuins are believed to underlie the healthful effects of calorie restriction, and of course, calorie restriction is strongly associated with an enhanced healthy lifespan. Indian researchers published some research recently that showed that resveratrol helps quell potentially damaging inflammation. Specifically, it prevented diabetic neuropathy, a painful condition that often occurs in long-term diabetics as a result of diabetes-induced nerve damage.

In their study, the Indian researchers reported that resveratrol inhibited one of the most damaging metabolic pathways involved in the inflammatory response, by targeting a compound called necrosis factor kappa beta (NF-kappaB). This is a key compound in the body's inflammatory cascade. This research indicated that resveratrol may help prevent the damage and deterioration associated with diseases that are considered inflammatory conditions. These include atherosclerosis and arthritis, among others.

The scientists reported that resveratrol also reduced levels of other inflammation-mediating molecules, including tumor necrosis factor-alpha (TNF-alpha), interleukin-6 and COX-2. COX-2 is a key inflammatory protein that is targeted by many modern anti-inflammatory medications, such as aspirin, ibuprofen and naproxen, which reduce pain and inflammation.

This ability of resveratrol to reduce inflammation through specific mechanisms of action was confirmed by Chinese researchers working in the laboratory with human cells. They were able to show that resveratrol modulates gene expression to reduce NF-kappa beta production. This research was especially illuminating, as it showed that resveratrol's beneficial effects are not solely dependent on its antioxidant activity. Rather, it also directly modifies the inflammatory cascade, which is involved in so many degenerative conditions.

SDG Lignans

Lignans are plant nutrients found in foods like flaxseed. These important phytonutrients may not be on the tip of everyone's tongue, but they probably should be. They've been credited with potent beneficial activities linked to cancer prevention and heart disease prevention.

In fact, animal study results prompted one scientist to declare that plant lignans have clear anticarcinogenic effects against numerous types of cancer. Lignans are among four classes of plant compounds collectively known as phytoestrogens. Chemically, they resemble estradiol, the most important of the estrogen hormones.

Although we think of estrogen as the "female hormone," both men and women have receptors for these hormones on tissues throughout the body. Some of these receptors are located on the linings of our arteries and in our brains, for example. These receptors are like miniature switches, which can be figuratively flipped on or off, either promoting or preventing certain cellular activities.

There are many plant lignans, but ultimately only two are of importance to human health. Plant lignans, such as SDG (secoisolariciresinol diglucoside) lignan (the primary lignan in healthful flaxseed), are converted in the gut into the so-called "mammalian lignans." Specifically, these are *enterolactone* and *enterodiol*; it is these two molecules that are biologically active within our bodies.

Research suggests that dietary plant phytoestrogens, such as SDG lignans, help regulate overall health after undergoing conversion to these biologically active compounds in the digestive tract. They accomplish their beneficial effects by working together with the body's own estrogen compounds to flip the right switches at the right times, so to speak.

Laboratory studies on animal models of human cancer have shown that dietary lignans inhibit or delay the growth of breast cancer, for example. Other experiments have yielded tantalizing evidence that lignans may protect against a wide variety of cancers, including liver, prostate, skin and colon cancers.

Of course, laboratory studies on animals and human cell cultures are considered preliminary, at best. But prospective studies on human subjects have strongly supported the notion that dietary lignan intake is associated with a reduced risk of breast cancer.

Given what we've learned so far about the links between plant-based diets and overall health, it should come as no surprise that many of the foods that typify a Mediterranean-type diet—whole grains, nuts, seeds, legumes, fruits, and vegetables—are rich sources of lignans. And like the Mediterranean diet itself, a high intake of lignans has been linked to a reduced risk of cardiovascular disease.

Ginger

Ginger (*Zingiber officinale*) has been prized as a culinary and medicinal herb for centuries, and it has long been believed to possess anti-diabetic properties. Scientists have confirmed that ginger contains potent anti-inflammatory compounds, called gingerols. And evidence obtained mostly from animal studies indicates that ginger improves blood lipid and triglyceride levels.

In laboratory animals fed a high-fat diet, plus ginger, ginger also reduced blood glucose, body weight, and insulin levels, compared to control animals that received a high-fat diet without ginger. As yet another example of the potential health benefits of this natural superfood, scientists also reported recently that ginger extract significantly reduced the occurrence of diabetes-induced cataracts in a rat model of human diabetes. This effect is apparently related to ginger's ability to discourage the formation of chemicals called advanced-glycation endproducts (AGEs).

The AGEs are a group of molecules formed when sugars react with free amino groups on proteins, lipids and nucleic acids. One example of this is hemoglobin A1C (HbA1C). This particular AGE is such a reliable indicator of uncontrolled high blood sugar that doctors often order this blood test on their patients who may be pre-diabetic or diabetic, as it provides a sort of snapshot of their patients' past few months of blood sugar levels. When HbA1C levels exceed 7%, doctors know that blood sugar control has become a problem.

Although monitoring of HbA1C is a useful diagnostic tool, its presence is highly undesirable. In fact, the AGEs are responsible for many of the complications associated with diabetes and its damage throughout the body. AGEs are even suspected of playing a role in many of the signs of aging, such as wrinkles, and cataracts. AGE formation is greatly enhanced by oxidative stress, which, as we've seen, results when free radicals overwhelm the body's supplies of antioxidants, both naturally generated and obtained through the diet. Ginger supplies some of the antioxidant boost needed to prevent oxidative stress.

Quercetin

Quercetin is a natural flavonoid compound. It is abundant in plant foods such as onions and apples. As it turns out, quercetin may well be the reason the old adage, "An apple a day keeps the doctor away," is a wise saying. Scientists are actively studying quercetin's many benefits, which evidently stem from its antioxidant and anti-inflammatory effects in the body.

According to a study published in the *British Journal of Nutrition*, supplementation with quercetin decreased oxidized LDL-cholesterol and lowered blood pressure in overweight people who were at risk of developing cardiovascular disease.

The subjects in this well-controlled trial received 150 mg of quercetin every day, or an inactive placebo, for six weeks. After a five-week washout period, the subjects were switched to the alternate treatment. Neither investigators nor subjects knew who was receiving which substance. Researchers measured the subjects' blood pressure and blood lipid profiles after each phase of the trial.

Subjects with high blood pressure experienced a decrease in systolic blood pressure while taking quercetin, but not while taking the placebo. In a subgroup of adults aged 25-50 years, quercetin supplementation resulted in an even greater drop in systolic blood pressure. Quercetin also significantly decreased concentrations of oxidized LDL-cholesterol, which plays a key role in the development of atherosclerosis.

Quercetin is also credited with potent anticancer activities. In addition to its powerful antioxidant activity, which is believed to underlie some of its anticancer benefits, quercetin also exerts a direct anti-tumor effect that is independent of this antioxidant activity. Laboratory studies have shown that it is capable of blocking the growth of several cancer cell types at various phases of the cells' growth cycles.

Plant Enzymes and Fibers

My formulas contain various natural enzymes that are found either in our digestive systems, or in some of the plants we eat, or both. All of these enzymes help us break down various components of our food in the digestive tract, so that we can benefit from food's full nutritional value.

Protease, for example, is an enzyme that helps break down proteins into their constituent amino acids, while lipase is an enzyme that breaks down fats, helping release their energy.

Lactase helps the body break down lactose (milk sugar) from dairy products, and cellulase can help prevent a rare condition called gastric phytobezoar, in which undigested cellulose, or plant fiber, forms a mass with other plant constituents, potentially causing blockage within the gastrointestinal system.

Among the various enzymes included in my Plant Enzyme and Fiber blends, I also include oat bran. Oat bran is a natural compound largely responsible for oatmeal's well-deserved reputation as a heart-healthy food. That's because these mostly indigestible, soluble fibers help lower cholesterol levels, among other activities.

Although they are non-digestible carbohydrates, they are considered to be physiologically beneficial. And that may be something of an understatement. It's not entirely clear how oat beta glucans found in oat bran help remove cholesterol from the bloodstream, but it's certain that they do.

In fact, due to the presence of beta glucans in oatmeal, manufacturers of the popular breakfast food are allowed, by law, to include statements on their packaging to the effect that eating oatmeal may help reduce the risk of heart disease. Few foods have jumped through enough hoops to have earned the right to make such a claim.

Studies have shown that diets high in oat beta glucans may yield significant reductions in "bad" LDL-cholesterol levels. What's more, in some individuals, oat beta glucan consumption has been linked to elevated levels of "good" HDL-cholesterol, which may be just as important for heart health as low "bad" cholesterol. Furthermore, oat beta glucans found in natural oat bran have been shown to improve blood sugar control, possibly by delaying stomach emptying, or by slowing uptake of glucose from the small intestines.

As if that's not enough evidence for the health benefits of this whole grain component, research shows that oat beta glucans can also significantly reduce blood pressure among obese people. This information was obtained from a well-controlled clinical trial.

Subjects were randomly selected to consume either oat beta glucans, or a placebo substance, for three months. Subjects who consumed oat beta glucans experienced significant blood pressure reductions, while control subjects who did not get the beta glucans did not experience these improvements. Tellingly, peak insulin levels also declined among subjects who consumed oat beta glucans. As we've already seen, dramatic spikes in glucose and insulin are hallmarks of prediabetes and diabetes.

Dairy Free Probiotics

Bacteria usually get a bad rap. After all, plenty of bacteria species cause harm. Some of the most feared diseases in history have been caused by bacteria. The Black Death, widely attributed to infection by the *Yersinia pestis* organism, killed nearly a third of the world's population in the fourteenth century. No one is likely to embrace the organism responsible for bubonic plague any time soon. So it's understandable that bacteria could benefit from a public relations makeover.

But it would be a mistake to lump all bacteria together, just because of a few bad apples. The fact is, bacteria can be—and in fact, often are—our friends. Emerging understanding of the inextricable relationships among humans and their resident bacteria is shedding new light on just how indispensable bacteria are in our everyday lives. To put it simply, many bacteria are not only harmless, they're highly beneficial. Mutually beneficial, symbiotic relationships between humans and certain types of "friendly" bacteria have been with us from the beginning.

We enter the world with sterile bodies, but beneficial bacteria quickly colonize the sites where the body "interfaces" with the environment, including the mouth, digestive tract and, in women, the vagina. This colonization is natural and helpful. Beneficial bacteria become established and quickly begin helping us in numerous ways. These include fighting off colonization by less benign organisms through a variety of mechanisms, and helping with digestion. For instance, colonization by friendly bacteria in the digestive tract helps to maintain the intestinal lining.

Relatively new evidence shows that friendly microorganisms even contribute to immunity. In the gut, bacteria contribute generously to the body's crucial supply of vitamin K. This vitamin is an essential lipid-soluble vitamin that plays a vital role in blood clotting. Beneficial bacteria, such as the species found in many types of live-culture yogurts, are believed to help aid digestion, and prevent infection with unfriendly microorganisms.

And that's why I also include oral probiotics in my formulas; probiotics are live microorganisms that benefit their hosts. Research suggests that probiotics may help alleviate chronic intestinal inflammatory conditions, and prevent diarrhea linked to disease-causing organisms (pathogens).

When people are required to take antibiotics, their colonies of beneficial bacteria (the intestinal microflora) often suffer. It is believed that consuming probiotics during and after a course of antibiotic therapy may help these beneficial bacteria re-colonize the gut, ensuring ongoing optimal digestive and immune system health.

Some strains of probiotics, such as *Lactobacillus bulgaricus*, have been shown in laboratory studies to reduce the damaging effects of food-borne carcinogens, such as heterocyclic amines. Other studies suggest that probiotics may help reduce serum cholesterol levels, and boost immune system function.

Interested in learning more about research that supports other ingredients I use in my powder mixes? Visit my website. In the *Reports* window, enter the key words "Ingredient Benefits" to download a free report on studies about individual ingredients.

A Work In Progress

Many years have passed since I first started formulating my products. My skill at creating new formulas that balance functionality with pleasing flavor has matured over time, just as the demand for new tastes has grown over the years.

My first formula was Delicious Greens "Original." I called it original because the flavor is unique. Some users describe it as minty; others say it tastes of cinnamon, while others find that it tastes like fresh tea. Still others describe it as redolent of orange blossoms, with a hint of licorice. The unique, almost impressionistic nature of the flavor arises from the unique combination of the various ingredients I use. All of my power mixes are Vegan, 100% natural, or Certified Organic, and they not only taste good, but they are good for you too.

Visit my website, CocoMarch.com, and click under *products* to learn more. You will find that over the years I have released a variety of flavors and blends, ranging from exotic fruity ones like Berry and Strawberry Kiwi, to more delicate ones like Silk Chocolate. My chocolate mix is very popular among parents, as well as children. Mixed in any type of milk, it tastes like cocoa. I also created a Mocha Greens Mix. It's made with dozens of different fruits and vegetables, but has no added caffeine beyond the small amount naturally present in the cocoa powder I use to make it brown instead of green. It truly tastes like one of those expensive coffee-shop concoctions. Who knew you could get your shot of veggies for the day so easily?

Most people can't wrap their heads around the variety of flavors I've created, but I guarantee you will be fully satisfied when you try any of my blends. Despite the success of my products, I have never abandoned the original mission: to create an ideal nutritional supplement in convenient powder form, which hews as closely to nature as possible and has a pleasant flavor. I've never given in to pressure to cut corners on ingredients. I continue to use only the highest-quality premium ingredients.

Even though my *Delicious Greens* and *Dr. Cocó Organics* lines are the best on the market, they are also the most affordable. I believe it's my life's purpose to make a difference. I also believe that if you're going to make a difference, you need to make what you have to offer available to as many people as possible.

My products are affordable because we choose affordability over profit. As I continue creating new, unique powder mixes of natural antioxidants and phytonutrients, I can assure you I'll faithfully continue to keep my products 100% natural, with no fillers and no artificial anything. And they'll continue to taste great!

You can learn more about my product lines by visiting my website at www.CocoMarch.com and clicking under the *Products* tab.

Real Fruit Vitamins

Earlier we talked about the benefits of antioxidants. Antioxidants are an important group of nutrients that are generally different from minerals and certain vitamins (although some vitamins and minerals may act as antioxidants in the body).

As you learned, just as the components of food can be divided into groups such as carbohydrates, proteins or fats, "micronutrients" and "macronutrients" are also divided into groups. Antioxidants are important components of a balanced diet. Some additional nutrients, such as magnesium (an essential mineral) and vitamin D (a natural hormone-like vitamin) should be enhanced by supplementing with a multivitamin that features minerals and vitamin D3.

My Greens line provides you with antioxidants but not with enough vitamins and minerals. As I said before and told my patients, you should supplement with a vita-mineral complex. To ensure you have a full spectrum of nutrients.

When I searched for a good multivitamin, I faced a similar problem as I did when I looked for a good antioxidant supplement. Most vitamins are simply made too cheaply. I told you before what I found when I looked at popular brands such as One a Day or Centrum. They all contain fillers and artificial ingredients, and the pills are often too large to swallow easily. And impossible to absorb.

To fill this small need, I created Real Fruit Vitamins; the only 100% natural fruit-based, powdered multivitamin. Real Fruit Vitamins is made with amazing ingredients. Each daily serving provides you with optimal levels of all necessary vitamins as well as minerals. Real Fruit Vitamins taste great and will help you achieve adequate levels of vitamins A, D,

E and K, as well as B vitamins and necessary minerals, such as calcium, magnesium, zinc, and chromium, among others.

My vitamins contain no fillers and no artificial ingredients. Instead, they contain a base of over 30 different fruits, plus 23 Immune Supporting Ingredients, such as bee pollen, royal jelly, and green tea, to mention a few. I am very proud of this formulation: There is no other like it. I wish I could recommend that you compare Real Fruit Vitamins to competitor's vitamins, but the truth is there is no comparison. If the quality and ingredients aren't enough to convince you that Real Fruit Vitamins are superior, there's always the taste. It tastes great!

You can visit my website, CocoMarch.com, to learn more or download a list of ingredients and benefits from included plants. Following is a list of the ingredients in one daily serving of Real Fruit Vitamins.

DR. MARCH'S 30 FRUITS VITA-BLEND

ORGANIC STRAWBERRY FRUIT POWDER
ORGANIC BANANA FRUIT POWDER
ORGANIC RASPBERRY FRUIT POWDER
ORGANIC RED APPLE FRUIT POWDER
ORGANIC GREEN APPLE FRUIT POWDER
ORGANIC RED RASPBERRY FRUIT POWDER
ORGANIC BLACKBERRY FRUIT POWDER
ORGANIC CABBAGE PALM FRUIT POWDER (Açaí)
ORGANIC BLACK RASPBERRY FRUIT POWDER
ORGANIC BLUEBERRY FRUIT POWDER
ORGANIC CANTALOUPE POWDER
ORGANIC ELDERBERRY POWDER
ORGANIC LYCIUM BERRY POWDER (GOJI)
ORGANIC GRAPE JUICE POWDER
ORGANIC KIWI FRUIT POWDER
ORGANIC LEMON JUICE POWDER
NONI JUICE POWDER
ORGANIC POMEGRANATE FRUIT POWDER
APRICOT KERNELS FRUIT POWDER
MANGO FRUIT POWDER

MANGOSTEEN FRUIT POWDER
MAQUI BERRY FRUIT POWDER
ORANGE FRUIT POWDER
PAPAYA FRUIT POWDER
PEAR FRUIT POWDER
PINEAPPLE FRUIT POWDER
PLUM FRUIT POWDER
ORGANIC BARBADOS CHERRY ACEROLA
RED GRAPE SEED EXTRACT 4:1
WATERMELON FRUIT POWDER

DR.MARCH'S IMMU-AID BLEND
RED BEET ROOT POWDER
ORGANIC CARROT ROOT POWDER
VEGETABLE & FRUIT ANTIOXIDANT BLEND
PURPLE CABBAGE LEAVES POWDER
GREEN TEA LEAF EXTRACT (Decaf.)
POMEGRANATE FRUIT EXTRACT 4:1
TURMERIC ROOT POWDER
ATLANTIC KELP POWDER
JAPANESE KNOTWEED ROOT EXTRACT
POLYGONUM CUSPIDATUM (TRANS RESVERATROL)
GRAPE PEEL EXTRACT (RED WINE EXTRACT)
ORGANIC ALOE VERA LEAF POWDER
ORGANIC BROCCOLI JUICE POWDER
ORGANIC CAULIFLOWER JUICE POWDER
ORGANIC SPINACH JUICE POWDER
ORGANIC PARSLEY JUICE POWDER
MILK THISTLE SEED EXTRACT
BLACK RADISH POWDER
OMEGA-3 CHIA SEED
BROWN RICE BRAN
BEE POLLEN POWDER
ROYAL JELLY POWDER
GINKGO BILOBA LEAF POWDER

The Panacea?

I would love to tell you that my inventions are a panacea; the cure for all diseases. But I would never do that. And I would never tell you to substitute taking any of my Delicious Greens or Real Fruit Vitamins products for following my True Nutrition Plan and eating a variety of organic fruits and vegetables every day.

My powder mixes Delicious Greens and Real Fruit Vitamins are supplements. Supplement means enhancement; in addition to, not panacea.

I want you to focus on eating right as I have taught you in this book. Your lifestyle is key to your success. Don't feel you can just take my products and feel great forever while continuing to do what you have been doing so far. Taking my products alone will certainly make you feel better, there is no doubt about it. But True Nutrition is not about feeling a little bit better. It is about giving your body the tools it needs to correct your health and feel great and vibrant forever.

In fact, if you can eat plenty of organic fruits and vegetables on a daily basis, you don't really need to use my products, because you will be getting most of you nutrition that way. But if you can only eat some fruits and vegetables, I highly encourage you to supplement with my formulas. Notice I said *supplement*; you still need to make an effort to increase your produce consumption. Do not rely on just Delicious Greens and Real Fruit Vitamins to get your recommended servings of fruits and vegetables. Fresh, whole foods from nature are always best.

Secrets to remember:

- The Dr. Coco's product line supplies natural enzymes, trace minerals, probiotics, fiber, phytonutrients, and powerful antioxidants equivalent to as many as 20 servings of fruits and vegetables in each serving.
- Delicious Greens is not a multivitamin. It is not intended to replace your daily multivitamin supplement.
- Lifestyle is crucial to success. Don't feel you can just take my products and feel great forever while continuing to do what you have been doing so far.

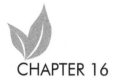

CHAPTER 16

Take Action

An ounce of action is worth a ton of theory.
Ralph Waldo Emerson

I f you are a parent, you're almost certainly aware that toddlers start asking questions soon after they utter their first words. You also know that your initial answer is seldom sufficient. Little ones frequently want to know more. "Why" seems to be a particular favorite. As we grow up we stop asking as many questions. Often, some of the most important questions go unasked—and unanswered—and "why" is one of them.

When it comes to your health you need to know *why* you're making certain choices or changes. Understanding the why of change moves your new behavior out of the realm of fad, and into the realm of lifestyle—and hopefully, lifetime—change. I have spent countless years researching and polishing this plan. In the previous chapters you learned what happens if you simply continue eating the way most Americans do. You now also know the many benefits of following My True Nutrition Plan to feel better and reach optimal weight. True Nutrition is not a diet; it's a lifestyle. Understanding and remembering "why" you have made changes to adopt healthy new habits will help you avoid settling back into old routines, which may lead to choices you don't want to revisit.

I encourage you to read and study this book from beginning to end, a couple times per year. As we say in Spain, "La repetición es la madre de la retención". This roughly translates to the idea that you need to repeat things in order to avoid forgetting them (literally: Repetition is the mother of retention). You now have the foundation for success; the power to overcome the temptation of not living and eating the True Nutrition way.

Breakfast

A recent survey by the NPD Group found that 31 million Americans—that's about 10 percent of the U.S. population—do not eat breakfast. The most common reasons people gave for skipping breakfast were: they weren't hungry, they didn't feel like eating, or they were too busy.

Breakfast is the most important meal of the day. Remember that you haven't eaten while resting, so your body is ready for refueling. In my experience, many people are too busy to think much about breakfast and end up grabbing something less than healthy on the go. Or they eat nothing at all.

I agree that we are all busy. And mornings are no different. For that reason, I suggest using breakfast solutions that are quick and easy for the whole family. Starting the day with protein is essential, and smoothies can be a simple breakfast approach for many on-the-go families. My easy Sinless Pudding recipe can be prepared in a couple of minutes. It's great for quick snacks, or days on-the-go. A serving of Protein Powder with Delicious Greens will also provide your body with the essentials you need. The key is to never start your day with an empty stomach.

Smoothies

To make smoothies you will need a blender. I have had a VitaMix blender for more than ten years. It's still churning out great drinks. This brand is rather expensive (usually around $400.00), so if your budget doesn't allow for a VitaMix, start with a more economical model. I've also used the Magic Bullet for one-person shakes. It's small and convenient and can be a good place to start. But if smoothies become part of your family's routine, a more powerful blender may be a better investment. Larger blenders allow you to mix enough for everyone all at once, which is far more convenient if you have a family of four or more.

Snacks

Snacks anyone? Why not? True Nutrition works best when you feed your body every two to three hours. Snacking is a great way to avoid overeating at lunch and dinner time. It also ensures that you're giving your body smaller portions of food that it can readily digest. Chew slowly and take your time. Some of the best snacks for curbing hunger and protecting your heart are nuts like almonds, cashews, hazelnuts, macadamia nuts, or peanuts. Organic Cheese Sticks, organic whole-wheat crackers, apples, and carrots are all good snacks, too.

Lunch

I think eating out for lunch is one of the biggest mistakes you can make. Eating out is not only expensive, it's also likely to involve food that's high in calories. It's true that in Spain, and most other Mediterranean countries, we typically eat a large lunch. But there's a distinct cultural difference. In the Mediterranean, lunch is the main meal of the day. Dinner is a modest meal for the majority of Mediterranean families. Most suppers consist of some fresh fruit, or snacking on a few things; not a large meal. In the U. S., though, people routinely go out for lunch and feast, easily consuming more than 1,000 calories. Then they go home and have an even larger meal for dinner.

Even if it's a quick lunch, most restaurant meals are far from healthy, and they're invariably expensive. And don't get me started on fast food. These "restaurants" offer the epitome of bad choices. I suggest taking your lunch from home. It will help you trim your body as well as your budget. It also allows you to control what you are eating at a fraction of the cost of dining out. Whether you are trying to lose weight or not, any of the lunch options in the Sinless Diet section are good. They're full of nutrients and easy to make.

Dinner

This is not a recipe book, but you will find a number of dinner recipes at the end of this book. I've collected a few that are fast, easy, and healthy. Most recipes take 30 minutes or less. They're examples of how easy it is to make healthy meals if you just plan ahead.

Drink

You've heard it before, but I'll repeat it here: Drink water. Plenty of water. If you are trying to lose weight, I recommend drinking one ounce of water per day for each pound of body weight. Everyone else should aim for about seven fluid ounces of water for every 10 pounds of body weight. Make sure your water is filtered. Later I'll talk about the benefits of owning a reverse osmosis water purification system.

I recommend that you avoid drinking while you are eating. Drinking too much while eating can dilute your digestive enzymes making digestion slower and more difficult. I recommend drinking a couple of large glasses of water ten or fifteen minutes before you start your meal. It will help you be less thirsty while eating. It will also encourage you to eat less.

Avoid using too much ice. Water should be your main drink every day, preferably without ice. Americans have a habit of filling their glasses with ice before adding their already-cold beverages. There is no need to add ice to cool water most of the time. According to the ancient Indian system of folk medicine, Ayurveda, drinking cold refreshments has a negative impact on digestion. Chinese doctors claim that regular consumption of iced drinks can play a role in female infertility as well as causing immune and digestive problems.

Avoid All Sodas

I probably don't need to tell you that sodas are bad. Any type of soda should be avoided. Sugary sodas have the same bad effects as diet sodas. Diet sodas have the benefit of not adding calories to your diet, but consuming harmful artificial sweeteners like aspartame or Sucralose (Splenda®) can cause numerous health problems.

Aspartame has been linked to many health problems, including brain tumors. In fact the father of a good friend of mine was recently operated on for a type of brain tumor called glioblastoma multiforme. There is no cure for it and it's very aggressive. Once it has been removed doctors can try to control the growth with radiation, but the prognosis is usually not good and most patients die within a few months or years.

When I went to visit him, his wife told me that he had always been healthy. In fact, he had been diabetic for several decades without suffering any side effects, which was considered rare for someone who's been using insulin for so long. "Because of his diabetes he never drank regular sodas, only diet, and he drank them frequently," she said. "We were told by a diabetes specialist decades ago that aspartame could cause brain tumors, but if he wanted to enjoy something sweet, he should avoid sugar and use aspartame instead."

Evidence now suggests that aspartame is dangerous just like saccharine, or sucralose. They are all chemicals that do not belong in the True Nutrition Lifestyle. To drink a diet soda once in a great while will not kill anyone. But drinking them with any regularity allows these foreign chemicals to accumulate in your system. What may hurt one person quickly may take decades to damage someone else, but the bottom line is that you are not doing yourself any good by consuming these artificial chemicals.

So why not just to get used to drinking water? You can add natural flavors, if you want. These are sold in liquid form, next to the spice rack in most groceries and health foods stores. Add to your water with a few drops of Stevia. Or you can add lemon juice and some Stevia for a tasty lemonade flavor.

Reverse Osmosis System (RO)

The more you drink water, the more appealing it becomes. As a child I did not love drinking water. But in my later years I became determined to drink it for my health. Initially it was difficult, but in time I fell in love with the taste. Particularly when I began drinking water that had been purified with an RO system.

While completing work on this book I was traveling from Minnesota to Barbados. On the first leg of my trip I happened to sit next to a gentleman named Peter Cartwright. After our four-hour conversation I renamed him the "Water Guru."

Peter is a Chemical Engineer. He works in Minnesota and Amsterdam, where he has an office. Peter travels the world, consulting, lecturing and writing hundreds of articles about the importance of water safety. I was so impressed by everything I learned from him that I felt compelled to share with you some of what he told me.

Peter mentioned that even though our city water is considered safe, there are benefits to owning an RO system for drinking water. "Although the drinking water quality requirements are met when the water leaves the treatment plants of most cities in the United States, this water may become contaminated traveling through the distribution system," he said.

According to the Water Guru, "If a consumer wants to take that extra step to ensure the delivery of high quality water, I suggest the installation of an under-sink reverse osmosis (RO) system in the home. This technology will produce an acceptable quality of drinking water."

When I asked him about more expensive systems, Mr. Cartwright replied: "A reverse osmosis system will produce the highest quality of drinking water for the price. It will remove a high percentage of dissolved salts and most organic compounds." Most RO systems on the market today include a carbon pre-filter to remove chlorine as well as sediments. This serves to protect the membrane, which is at the heart of the reverse osmosis process of filtration. After the membrane treatment, the water is further filtered through another carbon filter (post-treatment), which ensures that the water will have optimum taste.

This is basically triple filtration. "I am not aware of any system that does not use this arrangement" Cartwright said. According to him, a good recommendation is to purchase only a system that has been tested to meet the standards of NSF 58. This ensures that the unit will perform to meet rigid manufacturing and performance requirements.

Like many others, my family has its own well. Well water is assumed to be more or less pristine. However, according to Cartwright: "There is evidence that more and more wells are becoming contaminated, particularly as a result of industrial or agricultural activities nearby. This is particularly true for shallow wells, such as those less than 100 feet deep. Any well owner should be aware of nearby activity, and perhaps have the water analyzed every year, just to be safe.

Secrets to remember:

- Never start your day with an empty stomach. Breakfast is the most important meal of the day, and starting with protein is crucial.

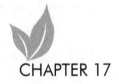

CHAPTER 17

Dr. Cocó's Sinless Diet

Some rise by sin, and some by virtue fall.
William Shakespeare

Having unrealistic goals will set you up for disappointment and failure. We're not going to let that happen. You are not alone. We are working together on your new eating habits. These habits are the key to your success, not only at losing weight, but at being healthy. What good is it to have be skinny if you are not feeling good enough to enjoy it? These new practices will provide you with nutritious foods that keep you healthy and help you lose weight at a steady, realistic pace.

Nevertheless, I realize that there may be a time when you need to shed a few pounds more quickly. I have created Dr. Coco's Sinless Diet for such situations. The Sinless Diet is a revolutionary new approach that helps you lose weight by balancing proteins, fats and carbohydrates the True Nutrition way. A couple of foods figure prominently in the Sinless Diet, because I recommend eating these foods once or more each day. These key Sinless Diet foods are yogurt and nuts.

Yogurt

I have mentioned yogurt a couple times already, and it bears repeating here because it's a key Sinless Diet food. I'm a personal fan of yogurt, but I want you to know that I don't just recommend it because I like it. There's actually scientific evidence that yogurt can play an important role in weight loss. For example, a recent study published in the *New England Journal of Medicine* suggests such a link between yogurt and weight loss. Conducted by the Harvard School of Public Health, the study's authors concluded that the regular consumption of yogurt and nuts had a positive impact on weight loss.

In a different study, supported by the Bell Institute of Health and Nutrition, researchers found that obese adults who ate three servings of fat-free yogurt a day as part of a reduced-calorie diet lost 22% more weight and 61% more body fat than those who simply cut calories and didn't increase their calcium intake with yogurt. Yogurt eaters also lost 81% more fat in the stomach area than non-yogurt eaters.

Nuts

Although high in fat, nuts are not fattening. Rather, they are a rich, nutritious, satisfying food that you can snack on regularly. Most nuts contain healthy various minerals, and unsaturated fats, which are known to help lower bad cholesterol levels. Some nuts, such as English walnuts, contain the healthful omega-3 fatty acid, alpha-linolenic acid (ALA). According to the Mayo Clinic's website, omega-3 fatty acids, "...seem to help your heart by, among other things, preventing dangerous heart rhythms that can lead to heart attacks". Nuts are also rich in fiber, vitamin E, plant sterols (which are also linked to lower "bad" LDL-cholesterol levels), and many other nutrients.

Walnuts are considered inflammation fighters. They are among the richest sources of the plant omega-3 fatty acid, ALA. They also contain the most antioxidants. Almonds contain the most fiber, and studies suggest they can play an important role in maintaining a healthy weight. In one study, published in the *International Journal of Obesity*, two groups of obese adults followed low-calorie diets for six months. Subjects who included almonds in their weight loss plans lost more weight than those who ate more complex carbohydrates. Cashews are known for their zinc content, which is critical for optimal immune system health. Pecans are my personal favorite, though.

A Balanced Approach

Unlike many popular plans, the Sinless Diet is a balanced regimen that allows you to eat satisfying portions of a variety of foods at regular intervals. Some of the options are so easy and delicious you'll feel you are committing a sin by eating them! But the truth is, it's all Sinless.

If you're like most American women, by now you've already tried dieting. With little or no success. High fat, low fat, high protein, no carbs; you name it. But the truth is, none of these fad diets make much sense, which is why they don't work in the long term. Your body needs reasonable amounts of food from all the food groups. A diet that splurges on one or two food groups, such as red meat and fat, while restricting carbs to nearly zero, is simply not realistic. It is also impractical, because you may be able to follow it briefly, but certainly not indefinitely.

By the same token, diets that require you to fast for days, or to limit your calorie intake to 500 calories a day, are just not reasonable. I do not recommend them. I am not saying you won't lose weight with these extreme types of diets. I am saying you will not be able to keep the weight off. Most people I have seen commit to such fad diets regained the weight as soon as they went back to eating normally.

Very low calorie diets (VLCD), where you consume just a few hundred calories per day, every day, for weeks, can certainly result in significant weight loss. But the cost is very high. With such diets, you are not teaching your body to be satisfied with reasonable amounts of food. You are simply not eating. The result is a potentially damaged metabolism, and rebound weight gain for most people.

Starving yourself is *not* the right way to lose weight. If you want to keep the weight off you simply must eat a balanced diet. This excludes any diet where you must nearly or totally eliminate an entire food group. Diets based on drinking juice or eating cookies, for example, simply don't work.

You must be real on your way to ideal.

My Sinless Diet Plan is designed to keep you feeling satisfied while losing weight and feeling healthier.

I have used the True Nutrition Approach, but factored in a schedule and carefully selected portions. Another important component of the Sinless Diet is to eat and drink at the proper times. I encourage you to drink plenty of water. Water helps your body in every sense, while helping you flush out the fat you are going to burn.

Drink *before* meals, but not *with* meals. Drinking 15 to 30 minutes before a meal gives your body the fluids it needs for easy digestion, while drinking during meals can dilute your digestive enzymes and make your digestion more difficult. Something else that I not only allow, but also recommend, is red wine. Have one small glass per day. Unlike water, it can be enjoyed with your dinner, or after.

Avoid soft drinks, even if they are diet beverages. We've already seen how unhealthy artificial sweeteners are. Sodas can be addictive, but I promise you that if you force yourself to drink water you will eventually love it. It takes effort to become accustomed to drinking plain water, but making the effort truly pays off.

Eating Frequently

The schedule I have made is hypothetical. Yours may start at 5 a.m., or 8 a.m., rather than 6:30 a.m. The intention is to illustrate the intervals that you should strive to maintain. Notice that you will be eating something every couple of hours. I want you to eat *even if you are not hungry*. That's very important. Stick as closely as you can to the schedule.

All the meals in the Sinless Diet are easy to make. I know your time is precious. If you are like me, you want this to be as simple as possible. In the Sinless Recipe section I describe in detail how to make anything that is not self-explanatory.

The recipes cover six days. Day 7 is Sinless Pudding Day. On Day 7 you'll have Sinless Pudding for breakfast, lunch and dinner, with a few healthy snacks in-between. Trust me, Sinless Pudding is delicious. The following week you start with Day 1 again. You can repeat this plan for as many weeks as you need until you reach your desired weight. It is inexpensive, healthy and easy to follow. And most importantly, it works.

To use organic ingredients in all your recipes is ideal, but if your budget doesn't allow it, replace organic ingredients with all-natural ones or conventional ingredients. For example I recommend Ezekiel Bread as your source of bread because it's organic, made with sprouted grains, and very filling. But if you don't like it, or can't afford it, choose a whole wheat bread with no sugars, honey or corn syrup. Be sure to read labels.

I don't have any affiliation with the makers of Ezekiel Bread, and I don't profit in any way if you purchase this or any other brand. When I make specific recommendations such as this, it's because I know the ingredients are wholesome and good for you and I have personally tried it, or use it regularly. If you are gluten intolerant chose gluten-free bread (also without sugars).

Coffee

I also list coffee as an optional drink for the morning; you can have one cup of coffee per day, or none. If drinking coffee first thing in the morning is not what you normally do, you can have it at a different time of day. If you don't drink coffee or tea then just skip these beverages altogether. Don't use any flavored creamers. You can, however, use plain half and half. But use no more than a couple tablespoons per cup of coffee.

Flaxseed

Flaxseed provides bulk and fiber, not to mention essential fatty acids. It's important to make sure your flaxseeds are ground. If not, you won't get the full benefit from this superfood, since the healthful oil will remain trapped inside. Flaxseed is inexpensive, and it's rather easy to find at most grocery and health food stores.

I recommend washing down flaxseed with plenty of water because a lot of people don't like having little seeds getting in between their teeth. But you can also chew it if you like the taste and the texture doesn't bother your teeth. Another option is to add it to your smoothies or salads. I find that taking it in the morning ensures you won't forget this important food, as it will quickly become a habit.

Dr. Cocó's 2-Day Prelude

If you are trying to lose weight, the 2-Day Prelude is an important step designed to prepare your body for weight loss.

You will lose weight over these two days because you will subject yourself to a liquid/vegetable fast. This initial weight loss is not from lost fat, however. It's mostly water. That's why I am don't believe in Very Low Calorie Diets or liquid diets. By following the 2-Day Prelude you will be cleansing your body while also shrinking the size of your stomach. This is a crucial step for a successful Sinless Diet.

You need only do the 2-Day Prelude when you begin the Sinless Diet. If you chose to follow my Sinless Plan for more than seven days, do not repeat the prelude; it's unnecessary.

Prelude Day One & Day Two

Vegetable Broth Unlimited, or Delicious Greens, or Dr. Cocó Organic Greens. The vegetable broth recipe is very simple. You'll find all the instructions at my website, CocoMarch.com. Enter the key words "Prelude vegetable broth" in the *Reports* search window to download free instructions for preparing the broth.

If you don't have time to make your own broth purchase one of my Delicious Greens formulas and use it mixed in water, following the instructions on the canister. During the Prelude you may chose to drink it cold or warm, as a broth or a tea, by mixing it in warm water.

You can drink as many servings and as much vegetable broth as you like. The purpose of this phase is to prepare for the Dr. Cocó's Sinless Diet.

Dr. Cocó's Sinless Diet

Day 1

6:30 a.m.	2-12 fl oz water
6:45 a.m.	Coffee or tea (cream & Stevia optional)
7:00 a.m.	2 Tbsp flaxseed (wash down with water or chew)
7:15 a.m.	Power House Smoothie Chocolate
9:00 a.m.	2-12 fl oz water
10:00 a.m.	1 small apple, well chewed
11:00 a.m.	2-12 fl oz water
12:00 p.m.	Creamy Tomato Turkey Ezekiel Sandwich
1:00 p.m.	2-12 fl oz of water
2:00 p.m.	12 almonds
3:00 p.m.	2-12 fl oz of water
4:00 p.m.	1 scoop of Delicious Greens in shaker cup
5:00 p.m.	2-12 fl oz of water
6:00 p.m.	Green salad
	Wild Smoked Alaskan Salmon with Rice
	4 fl oz glass of red wine or
	1 Flavored Greek Yogurt

Day 1: Recipes And Instructions

 Power House Smoothie

1 scoop Vanilla Protein Powder

1 Scoop Delicious Greens Chocolate

1/2 frozen banana

1 cup unsweetened almond milk

1/2 cup water

1/4 cup organic rolled oats

6 cubes ice

Put all ingredients in the blender, blend and drink.

 Creamy Tomato Turkey Sandwich

2 slices Ezekiel or whole-wheat bread

1 small tomato

1 Tbsp light cream cheese

3 slices turkey

Olive oil and salt

Cut tomato in half. Rub the inside pulp of one half of the tomato on one slice of bread. Repeat with other tomato half until both slices are soaked with tomato juice/pulp. Sprinkle salt and spray olive oil on both sides of the bread. Spread cream cheese on one of the slices of bread. Add turkey and enjoy.

Green Salad

2 cups lettuce (more if desired)

1 medium tomato

1/4 onion, sliced (optional)

1 Tbsp almond slices

1 Tbsp cranberries

1 Tbsp olive oil for dressing

1 Tbsp balsamic vinegar

Salt and pepper to taste

Mix all ingredient in a bowl. Sprinkle with salt and pepper to taste. Using a sprayer to spray olive oil evenly throughout the salad.

 ### Wild Smoked Alaskan Salmon with Basmati Rice

6 oz wild smoked Alaskan salmon (Costco)

1 Tbsp Boursin cheese

3 Tbsp stock

Salt and pepper to taste

1/2 cup cooked brown rice (Basmati or other)

1/2 tbsp olive oil

Heat up stock and warm up salmon in pan. Meanwhile, prepare brown rice. When rice is done, add ½ Tbsp Boursin cheese and ½ Tbsp olive oil, mixing well. Use the remaining Boursin cheese and olive oil to coat salmon fillet.

Day 2

6:30 a.m.	2-12 fl oz water
6:45 a.m.	Coffee or tea (cream optional)
7:00 a.m.	2 Tbsp flaxseed (wash down with water)
7:15 a.m.	Coco's Sinless Pudding
9:00 a.m.	2-12 fl oz water
10:00 a.m.	1 hardboiled egg sprinkled with salt & pepper; 12 cashew nuts
11:00 a.m.	2-12 fl oz water
12:00 p.m.	Ham & cream cheese sandwich
1:00 p.m.	2-12 fl oz of water
2:00 p.m.	1 small banana mashed with 1/2 tbsp peanut butter
3:00 p.m.	2-12 fl oz of water
4:00 p.m.	1 scoop of Delicious Greens in shaker cup
5:00 p.m.	2-12 fl oz of water
6:00 p.m.	Turkey wrap
	1 medium pear, peach or apple
	Glass of red wine

Day 2: Recipes And Instructions

 Sinless Pudding

1 cup plain Greek yogurt

4 Tbsp water

1 tsp of peanut butter

1 scoop Chocolate Delicious Greens

1 tsp honey

Mix ingredients in a bowl. Add more water for a silkier consistency.

 Ham & Cream Cheese Sandwich

2 slices Ezekiel or whole-wheat bread

1 small tomato

1 Tbsp light cream cheese

3 slices ham

olive oil and salt

Cut tomato in half. Rub the inside pulp of one tomato half on one slice of bread. Repeat with other tomato half until both slices are soaked with tomato juice/pulp. Sprinkle salt and spray olive oil on both slices of bread. Spread cream cheese on one of the slices of bread. Add ham and enjoy.

Turkey Wrap

(2) 8" whole wheat tortillas

2 Tbsp light cream cheese

4 ounces thinly sliced deli turkey breast

handful baby spinach

1/2 cup shredded cheese

1/2 diced tomato

1 Tbsp sour cream

Spread cream cheese on tortillas. Sprinkle garlic powder on top. Layer ingredients, dividing them between tortillas.Drizzle with sour cream and dressing. Roll up tightly.

Day 3

6:30 a.m.	2-12 fl oz water
6:45 a.m.	Coffee or tea (cream optional)
7:00 a.m.	2 Tbsp flaxseed (wash down with water)
7:15 a.m.	2 Egg Breakfast and 1 apple
9:00 a.m.	2-12 fl oz water
10:00 a.m.	1 Slice of Provolone Cheese, 6 whole-wheat crackers and 1 pear
11:00 a.m.	2-12 fl oz water
12:00 p.m.	Coco's Sinless Pudding
1:00 p.m.	2-12 fl oz of water
2:00 p.m.	12 raw almonds and 1 medium peach
3:00 p.m.	2-12 fl oz of water
4:00 p.m.	1 scoop Delicious Greens in shaker cup
5:00 p.m.	2-12 fl oz of water
6:00 p.m.	Green Salad and Hot Dog on whole wheat bun 5 Chocolate Raisins 7 Organic Animal Crackers (Trader Joe's) Or 4 fl oz glass of red wine

Day 3: Recipes And Instructions

 2-Egg Breakfast

2 eggs in omelette or scrambled

1/2 Tbsp olive oil from sprayer

1 slice Ezekiel bread

1 large tomato slice

1 medium apple

Spray pan with olive oil. Cook eggs. Serve on a slice of Ezekiel bread with the tomato slice seasoned with salt and oil.

 Sinless Pudding

1 cup plain Greek yogurt

4 Tbsp of water

1 tsp peanut butter

1 scoop Chocolate Delicious Greens

1 tsp of honey

Mix ingredients in a bowl, add more water for a silkier consistency.

Green Salad

2 cups lettuce (more if you want)

1 medium tomato

1/4 onion sliced (optional)

1 Tbsp almond slices

1 Tbsp cranberries

1 Tbsp olive oil for dressing

1 Tbsp balsamic vinegar

Salt and pepper to taste

Mix all ingredients in a bowl. Sprinkle salt and pepper to taste. Using a sprayer, spray olive oil evenly throughout salad.

 ### Hot Dog on whole wheat bun

Whole-wheat hot dog bun

Hot dog

½ Tbsp ketchup

½ tsp mustard

diced onions

relish

Heat 2 Tbsp vegetable broth in a medium size pan. When warm, immerse hot dog and allow to heat through. Can also be cooked on the grill. Build hot dog using the above ingredients.

Day 4

6:30 a.m.	2-12 fl oz water
6:45 a.m.	Coffee or tea (cream optional)
7:00 a.m.	2 Tbsp flaxseed (wash down with water)
7:15 a.m.	Citrus Berry Smoothie
9:00 a.m.	2-12 fl oz water
10:00 a.m.	1/2 banana, 12 Macadamia nuts
11:00 a.m.	2-12 fl oz water
12:00 p.m.	1-Coco's Sinless Pudding
1:00 p.m.	2-12 fl oz of water
2:00 p.m.	1 Slice of Ezekiel Bread
	1/2 banana smash and spread on Bread
	1 Tbsp of Peanut Butter
3:00 p.m.	2-12 fl oz of water
4:00 p.m.	1 scoop Delicious Greens mixed in water
5:00 p.m.	2-12 fl oz of water
6:00 p.m.	Green Salad & Tuna Crunch
	1 medium fruit or 1 cup of berries
	4 fl oz glass of red wine or
	1 Flavored Greek Yogurt

Day 4: Recipes And Instructions

 Citrus Berry Smoothie

1 scoop vanilla protein powder

1 scoop Delicious Greens Strawberry Kiwi

1/2 frozen banana

1 cup unsweetened almond milk

1/2 cup water

1 cup frozen berries (plus ice, optional)

1/2 tsp lemon oil flavoring (found in grocery spice aisle)

Put all ingredients in the blender and blend until smooth.

 Sinless Pudding

1 cup plain Greek yogurt

4 Tbsp of water

1 tsp peanut butter

1 scoop Chocolate Delicious Greens

1 tsp honey

Mix ingredients in a bowl. Add more water for a silkier consistency.

Green Salad

2 cups lettuce (more if desired)

1 medium tomato

1/4 onion, sliced (optional)

1 Tbsp almond slices

1 Tbsp cranberries

1 Tbsp olive oil for dressing

1 Tbsp balsamic vinegar

Salt and pepper to taste

Mix all ingredients in a bowl. Sprinkle with salt and pepper to taste. Using a sprayer, spray olive oil evenly throughout salad.

 ### Tuna Crunch

Wild Albacore tuna, canned in water

2 Tbsp light mayo

8 crackers

Mix all ingredients in a small bowl, spread tuna mix on crackers.

Day 5

6:30 a.m.	2-12 fl oz water
6:45 a.m.	Coffee or tea (cream optional)
7:00 a.m.	2 Tbsp ground flaxseed
7:15 a.m.	Coco's Sinless Pudding; one serving
9:00 a.m.	2-12 fl oz water
10:00 a.m.	1 cup strawberries, 24 hazelnuts
11:00 a.m.	2-12 fl oz water
12:00 p.m.	Ham & Cream Cheese Sandwich
1:00 p.m.	2-12 fl oz of water
2:00 p.m.	1 medium fruit
	2 slices turkey (1 oz)
	1 cheese stick
3:00 p.m.	2-12 fl oz of water
4:00 p.m.	1 scoop Delicious Greens or Reds mixed in water
5:00 p.m.	2-12 fl oz of water
6:00 p.m.	Dry Rubbed Chicken with Broccoli and Rice
	1 cup Brown Rice
	4 fl oz glass of red wine (optional), Store bought Greek yogurt

Day 5: Recipes And Instructions

 Sinless Pudding

1 cup plain Greek yogurt

4 Tbsp of water

1 tsp peanut butter

1 scoop Chocolate Delicious Greens

1 tsp honey

Mix ingredients in a bowl. Add more water for a silkier consistency.

 Ham & Cream Cheese Sandwich

2 slices Ezekiel or whole-wheat bread

1 small tomato

1 Tbsp light cream cheese

3 slices ham

olive oil and salt

Cut tomato in half. Rub the inside pulp of one tomato half on one slice of bread. Repeat with other tomato half until both slices are soaked with tomato juice/pulp. Sprinkle salt and spray olive oil on both slices of bread. Spread cream cheese on one of the slices of bread. Add ham and enjoy.

Dry Rubbed Chicken

8 oz boneless skinless chicken breast

spray of olive oil

1 Tbsp honey

1/4 Tbsp paprika

1/2 tsp garlic powder

1/2 tsp onion powder

1/8 tsp dry mustard

Mix all ingredients in a zip-lock bag. Shake bag, ensuring that chicken breast is coated with spices and honey.
TIP: For more intense flavor, store in fridge overnight.
Cook in oven at 375 degrees for 20 minutes.

 ### Broccoli and Rice

1 cup broccoli

1/2 cup brown rice

olive oil

garlic, salt, pepper

While Dry Rubbed Chicken is baking, steam 1 cup of broccoli florets and cook 1/2 cup of brown rice. Sprinkle garlic powder, salt and pepper over broccoli and rice. Spray with olive oil until it's all glazed. Serve with chicken.

Day 6

6:30 a.m.	2-12 fl oz water
6:45 a.m.	Coffee or tea (cream optional)
7:00 a.m.	2 Tbsp ground flaxseed
7:15 a.m.	2-Egg Breakfast
9:00 a.m.	2-12 fl oz water
10:00 a.m.	12 Brazil nuts, 1 medium piece of fruit
11:00 a.m.	2-12 fl oz water
12:00 p.m.	Creamy Tomato Turkey Sandwich
1:00 p.m.	2-12 fl oz of water
2:00 p.m.	1 Flavored Greek Yogurt
3:00 p.m.	2-12 fl oz of water
4:00 p.m.	1 scoop Delicious Greens or Reds mixed in water
5:00 p.m.	2-12 fl oz of water
6:00 p.m.	Soup & Salad, Power House or Citrus Smoothie

Day 6: Recipes And Instructions

 ## 2-Egg Breakfast

2 eggs in omelette, or scrambled

1/2 Tbsp olive oil from sprayer

1 slice Ezekiel bread

1 large slice tomato

1 medium apple

Spray olive oil in pan and cook eggs. Serve on a slice of Ezekiel bread with tomato slice. Season with salt and oil.

 ## Creamy Tomato Turkey Ezekiel Sandwich

2 slices Ezekiel or whole-wheat bread

1 small tomato

1 Tbsp light cream cheese

3 slices turkey

olive oil and salt

Cut tomato in half. Rub the inside pulp of one half of the tomato on one slice of bread. Repeat with other tomato half until both slices are soaked with tomato juice/pulp. Sprinkle salt and spray olive oil on both sides of the bread. Spread cream cheese on one of the slices of bread. Add turkey and enjoy.

Green Salad

2 cups lettuce (more if desired)

1 medium tomato

1/4 onion, sliced (optional)

1 Tbsp almond slices

1 Tbsp cranberries

1 Tbsp olive oil for dressing

1 Tbsp balsamic vinegar

salt and pepper

Mix all ingredients in a bowl. Sprinkle salt and pepper to taste. Using a sprayer, spray olive oil evenly throughout the salad.

 Chicken Soup

1 can store bought chicken soup

Warm up and serve. Enhance flavor by sprinkling with garlic powder and ground pepper.

Day 7

6:30 a.m.	2-12 fl oz water
6:45 a.m.	Coffee or tea (cream optional)
7:00 a.m.	2 Tbsp ground flaxseed
8:00 a.m.	Coco's Sinless Pudding; one serving
9:00 a.m.	2-12 fl oz water
10:00 a.m.	1 piece of fruit, 1 cheese stick, 12 nuts (almonds, cashews, pecans…)
11:00 a.m.	2-12 fl oz water
12:00 p.m.	Coco's Sinless Pudding; one serving
1:00 p.m.	2-12 fl oz of water
2:00 p.m.	12 pieces of nuts, 1 piece of fruit
3:00 p.m.	2-12 fl oz of water
4:00 p.m.	1 scoop Delicious Greens or Reds mixed in water
5:00 p.m.	2-12 fl oz of water
6:00 p.m.	Coco's Sinless Pudding; one serving

If you would like to receive these recipes in digital format so you can have them on your phone or tablet, visit my website at CocoMarch. com. In the Reports window enter the key words: Sinless Recipes. It has been very satisfying to write this book for you. I hope you feel inspired to live your life in an even healthier way. If you need support, join my Facebook page, Dr. Coco. I would love to hear your comments and feedback.

Dr. Coco's True Nutrition – Suggested Reading

Chapter 2

Bateman B, Warner JO, et al. The effects of a double blind, placebo controlled, artificial food colourings and benzoate preservative challenge on hyperactivity in a general population sample of preschool children. *Arch Dis Child.* 2004 Jun;89(6):506-11.

Finniss DG, Kaptchuk TJ, et al. Biological, clinical, and ethical advances of placebo effects. *Lancet.* 2010 Feb 20;375(9715):686-95.

Lidstone SC, Schulzer M, et al. Effects of expectation on placebo-induced dopamine release in Parkinson disease. *Arch Gen Psychiatry.* 2010 Aug;67(8):857-65.

Morton DL, Brown CA, et al. Cognitive changes as a result of a single exposure to placebo. *Neuropsychologia.* 2010 Jun;48(7):1958-64. Epub 2010 Mar 21.

Chapter 3

[No authors listed] Artificial food colouring and hyperactivity symptoms in children. *Prescrire Int.* 2009 Oct;18(103):215.

Davidson LE, Hudson R, et al. Effects of exercise modality on insulin resistance and functional limitation in older adults: a randomized controlled trial. *Arch Intern Med.* 2009 Jan 26;169(2):122-31.

Fombonne E. Epidemiology of pervasive developmental disorders. *Pediatr Res.* 2009 Jun;65(6):591-8.

He K, Du S, et al. Consumption of monosodium glutamate in relation to incidence of overweight in Chinese adults: China Health and Nutrition Survey (CHNS). *Am J Clin Nutr.* 2011 Jun;93(6):1328-36. Epub 2011 Apr 6.

He K, Zhao L, et al. Association of monosodium glutamate intake with overweight in Chinese adults: the INTERMAP Study. *Obesity (Silver Spring).* 2008 Aug;16(8):1875-80. Epub 2008 May 22.

Heidenreich PA, Trogdon JG, et al. Forecasting the future of cardiovascular disease in the United States: a policy statement from the American Heart Association. *Circulation.* 2011 Mar 1;123(8):933-44. Epub 2011 Jan 24.

Hogervorst JG, Schouten LJ, et al. Dietary **acrylamide** intake and the risk of renal cell, bladder, and prostate cancer. *Am J Clin Nutr.* May 2008; Vol. 87, No. 5: 1428-1438.

McCann D, Barrett A, et al. Food additives and hyperactive behaviour in 3-year-old and 8/9-year-old children in the community: a randomised, double-blinded, placebo-controlled trial. *Lancet.* 2007 Nov 3;370(9598):1560-7.

Naruszewicz M, Zapolska-Downar D, et al. Chronic intake of potato chips in humans increases the production of reactive oxygen radicals by leukocytes and increases plasma C-reactive protein: a pilot study. *Am J Clin Nutr.* 2009 Jan 21. [Epub ahead of print]

Nigg JT, Lewis K, et al. Meta-analysis of attention-deficit/hyperactivity disorder or attention-deficit/hyperactivity disorder symptoms, restriction diet, and synthetic food color additives. *J Am Acad Child Adolesc Psychiatry.* 2012 Jan;51(1):86-97.e8.

Shi Z, Luscombe-Marsh ND, et al. Monosodium glutamate is not associated with obesity or a greater prevalence of weight gain over 5 years: findings from the Jiangsu Nutrition Study of Chinese adults. *Br J Nutr.* 2010 Aug;104(3):457-63. Epub 2010 Apr 7.

Wang J, Sarnola K, et al. The metabolic syndrome predicts incident congestive heart failure: a 20-year follow-up study of elderly Finns. *Atherosclerosis.* 2010 May;210(1):237-42. Epub 2009 Nov 10.

Chapter 4

Biedermann S, Tschudin P, Grob K. Transfer of bisphenol A from thermal printer paper to the skin. *Anal Bioanal Chem*. 2010 Sep;398(1):571-6. Epub 2010 Jul 11.

Chen JQ, Brown TR, Russo J. Regulation of energy metabolism pathways by estrogens and estrogenic chemicals and potential implications in obesity associated with increased exposure to endocrine disruptors. *Biochim Biophys Acta*. 2009 Jul;1793(7):1128-43. Epub 2009 Apr 5.

Colón I, Caro D, et al. Identification of Phthalate Esters in the Serum of Young Puerto Rican Girls with Premature Breast Development. *Environ Health Perspect*. 2000; 108(9).

COUNCIL ON ENVIRONMENTAL HEALTH. Policy Statement—Chemical-Management Policy: Prioritizing Children's Health. Pediatrics 2011 : peds.2011-0523v1-peds.2011-0523.

Filippelli GM, Laidlaw MA. The elephant in the playground: confronting lead-contaminated soils as an important source of lead burdens to urban populations. *Perspect Biol Med*. 2010 Winter;53(1):31-45.

Grün F, Blumberg B. Endocrine disrupters as obesogens. *Mol Cell Endocrinol*. 2009 May 25;304(1-2):19-29. Epub 2009 Mar 9.

Grün F. Obesogens. *Curr Opin Endocrinol Diabetes Obes*. 2010 Oct;17(5):453-9.

Hiyama M, Choi EK, et al. Bisphenol-A (BPA) Affects Reproductive Formation across Generations in Mice. *J Vet Med Sci*. 2011 May 2. [Epub ahead of print]

Kirchner S, Kieu T, et al. Prenatal exposure to the environmental obesogen tributyltin predisposes multipotent stem cells to become adipocytes. *Mol Endocrinol*. 2010 Mar;24(3):526-39. Epub 2010 Feb 16.

Krishnan AV, Stathis P, et al. Bisphenol-A: an estrogenic substance is released from polycarbonate flasks during autoclaving. *Endocrinology*. 1993 Jun;132(6):2279-86.

Le HH, Carlson EM, et al. Bisphenol A is released from polycarbonate drinking bottles and mimics the neurotoxic actions of estrogen in developing cerebellar neurons. *Toxicol Lett*. 2008 Jan 30;176(2):149-56. Epub 2007 Nov 19.

Loganathan SN, Kannan K. Occurrence of Bisphenol A in Indoor Dust from Two Locations in the Eastern United States and Implications for Human Exposures. *Arch Environ Contam Toxicol.* 2011 Jan 8. [Epub ahead of print]

Mahaffey KR, Clickner RP, Jeffries RA. Adult women's blood mercury concentrations vary regionally in the United States: association with patterns of fish consumption (NHANES 1999-2004). *Environ Health Perspect.* 2009 Jan;117(1):47-53. Epub 2008 Aug 25.

McKelvey W, Gwynn RC, et al. A biomonitoring study of lead, cadmium, and mercury in the blood of New York city adults. *Environ Health Perspect.* 2007 Oct;115(10):1435-41.

Mycyk M, Hryhorczuk D, Amitai Y. (2005). "Lead". In Erickson, TB; Ahrens, WR; Aks, S; Ling, L. *Pediatric Toxicology: Diagnosis and Management of the Poisoned Child.* McGraw-Hill Professional.

Chapter 5

Basciano H, Federico L, Adeli K. Fructose, insulin resistance, and metabolic dyslipidemia. *Nutr Metab (Lond).* 2005 Feb 21;2(1):5.

Choi HK, Willett W, Curhan G. Fructose-rich beverages and risk of gout in women. *JAMA.* 2010 Nov 24;304(20):2270-8. Epub 2010 Nov 10.

Marriott BP, Cole N, Lee E. National estimates of dietary fructose intake increased from 1977 to 2004 in the United States. *J Nutr.* 2009 Jun;139(6):1228S-1235S. Epub 2009 Apr 29.

Nseir W, Nassar F, Assy N. Soft drinks consumption and nonalcoholic fatty liver disease. *World J Gastroenterol.* 2010 Jun 7;16(21): 2579-88.

Ouyang X, Cirillo P, et al. Fructose consumption as a risk factor for non-alcoholic fatty liver disease. *J Hepatol.* 2008 Jun;48(6):993-9. Epub 2008 Mar 10.

Preiss D, Sattar N. Non-alcoholic fatty liver disease: an overview of prevalence, diagnosis, pathogenesis and treatment considerations. *Clin Sci (Lond).* 2008 Sep;115(5):141-50.

Smith MD, Asche F, et al. Food safety. Genetically modified salmon and full impact assessment. *Science.* 2010 Nov 19;330(6007):1052-3.

Sui X, Church TS, et al. Uric acid and the development of metabolic syndrome in women and men. *Metabolism.* 2008 Jun;57(6):845-52.

Tappy L, Lê KA. Metabolic effects of fructose and the worldwide increase in obesity. *Physiol Rev.* 2010 Jan;90(1):23-46.

Taylor EN, Curhan GC. Fructose consumption and the risk of kidney stones. *Kidney Int.* 2008 Jan;73(2):207-12. Epub 2007 Oct 10.

Thuy S, Ladurner R, et al. Nonalcoholic fatty liver disease in humans is associated with increased plasma endotoxin and plasminogen activator inhibitor 1 concentrations and with fructose intake. *J Nutr.* 2008 Aug;138(8):1452-5.

Tomiyama H, Higashi Y, et al. Relationships Among Hyperuricemia, Metabolic Syndrome, and Endothelial Function. Am J Hypertens. 2011 Apr 14. [Epub ahead of print]

Chapter 6

Aiello AE, Coulborn RM, et al. Effect of hand hygiene on infectious disease risk in the community setting: a meta-analysis. *Am J Public Health.* 2008 Aug;98(8):1372-81. Epub 2008 Jun 12.

Begley TH, White K, et al. Perfluorochemicals: potential sources of and migration from food packaging. *Food Addit Contam.* 2005 Oct;22(10):1023-31.

Billionnet C, Gay E, et al. Quantitative assessments of indoor air pollution and respiratory health in a population-based sample of French dwellings. *Environ Res.* 2011 Apr;111(3):425-34.

Blackmore-Prince C, Harlow SD, et al. Chemical hair treatments and adverse pregnancy outcome among Black women in central North Carolina. *Am J Epidemiol.* 1999 Apr 15;149(8):712-6.

Butt CM, Berger U, et al. Levels and trends of poly- and perfluorinated compounds in the arctic environment. *Sci Total Environ.* 2010 Jul 1;408(15):2936-65. Epub 2010 May 20.

Coronado M, De Haro H, et al. Estrogenic activity and reproductive effects of the UV-filter oxybenzone (2-hydroxy-4-methoxyphenyl-methanone) in fish. *Aquat Toxicol.* 2008 Nov 21;90(3):182-7. Epub 2008 Sep 10.

Crinnion WJ. The CDC fourth national report on human exposure to environmental chemicals: what it tells us about our toxic burden and how it assist environmental medicine physicians. *Altern Med Rev.* 2010 Jul;15(2):101-9.

Cui L, Zhou QF, et al. Studies on the toxicological effects of PFOA and PFOS on rats using histological observation and chemical analysis. *Arch Environ Contam Toxicol.* 2009 Feb;56(2):338-49. Epub 2008 Jul 26.

Houde M, Martin JW, et al. Biological monitoring of polyfluoroalkyl substances: A review. *Environ Sci Technol.* 2006 Jun 1;40(11): 3463-73.

Jensen AA, Leffers H. Emerging endocrine disrupters: perfluoroalkylated substances. *Int J Androl.* 2008 Apr;31(2):161-9.

Kantiani L, Llorca M, et al. Emerging food contaminants: a review. *Anal Bioanal Chem.* 2010 Nov;398(6):2413-27. Epub 2010 Jul 31.

Kunz PY, Fent K. Multiple hormonal activities of UV filters and comparison of in vivo and in vitro estrogenic activity of ethyl-4-aminobenzoate in fish. *Aquat Toxicol.* 2006 Oct 12;79(4):305-24. Epub 2006 Jun 30.

Naya T, Hosomi N, et al. Smoking, fasting serum insulin, and obesity are the predictors of carotid atherosclerosis in relatively young subjects. *Angiology.* 2007 Dec-2008 Jan;58(6):677-84.

Potera C. Smoking and secondhand smoke. Study finds no level of SHS exposure free of effects. *Environ Health Perspect.* 2010 Nov;118(11):A474.

Schebb NH, Inceoglu B, et al. Investigation of human exposure to triclocarban after showering and preliminary evaluation of its biological effects. *Environ Sci Technol.* 2011 Apr 1;45(7):3109-15. Epub 2011 Mar 7.

Schecter A, Päpke O, et al. Polybrominated diphenyl ether flame retardants in the U.S. population: current levels, temporal trends, and comparison with dioxins, dibenzofurans, and polychlorinated biphenyls. *J Occup Environ Med.* 2005 Mar;47(3):199-211.

Sinclair E, Mayack DT, et al. Occurrence of perfluoroalkyl surfactants in water, fish, and birds from New York State. *Arch Environ Contam Toxicol.* 2006 Apr;50(3):398-410. Epub 2006 Jan 24.

Suja F, Pramanik BK, Zain SM. Contamination, bioaccumulation and toxic effects of perfluorinated chemicals (PFCs) in the water environment: a review paper. *Water Sci Technol.* 2009;60(6): 1533-44.

Tao L, Kannan K, et al. Perfluorinated compounds in human milk from Massachusetts, U.S.A. *Environ Sci Technol.* 2008 Apr 15;42(8):3096-101.

Zhu LY, Lin JH. [Pollution trend and environmental behavior of perfluorooctanoic acid: a review]. *Ying Yong Sheng Tai Xue Bao.* 2008 May;19(5):1149-57.

Chapter 7

Azadbakht L, Esmaillzadeh A. Red meat intake is associated with metabolic syndrome and the plasma C-reactive protein concentration in women. *J Nutr.* 2009 Feb;139(2):335-9. Epub 2008 Dec 11.

Caselli G, Vallin J, et al. Age-specific mortality trends in France and Italy since 1900: period and cohort effects. *Eur J Popul.* 1987 Nov;3(1):33-60.

Esposito K, Maiorino MI et al. Prevention and control of type 2 diabetes by Mediterranean diet: a systematic review. *Diabetes Res Clin Pract.* 2010 Aug;89(2):97-102. Epub 2010 May 23.

Farajian P, Risvas G, et al. Very high childhood obesity prevalence and low adherence rates to the Mediterranean diet in Greek children: The GRECO study. *Atherosclerosis.* 2011 Apr 13. [Epub ahead of print]

Ferri C, Croce G, et al. C-reactive protein: interaction with the vascular endothelium and possible role in human atherosclerosis. *Curr Pharm Des.* 2007;13(16):1631-45.

Itsiopoulos C, Brazionis L, et al. Can the Mediterranean diet lower HbA1c in type 2 diabetes? Results from a randomized cross-over study. *Nutr Metab Cardiovasc Dis.* 2010 Jul 29.

Miyagi S, Iwama N, et al. Longevity and diet in Okinawa, Japan: the past, present and future. *Asia Pac J Public Health.* 2003;15 Suppl:S3-9.

Prior RL, Gu L, et al. Plasma antioxidant capacity changes following a meal as a measure of the ability of a food to alter in vivo antioxidant status. *J Am Coll Nutr.* 2007 Apr;26(2):170-81.

Salas-Salvadó J, Bulló M, et al. Reduction in the Incidence of Type 2-Diabetes with the Mediterranean Diet: Results of the PREDIMED-Reus Nutrition Intervention Randomized Trial. *Diabetes Care.* 2010 Oct 13. [Epub ahead of print]

Simopoulos AP. Human requirement for N-3 polyunsaturated fatty acids. *Poult Sci.* 2000 Jul;79(7):961-70.

Trichopoulou A, Bamia C, Trichopoulos D. Anatomy of health effects of Mediterranean diet: Greek EPIC prospective cohort study. *BMJ.* 2009 Jun 23;338:b2337.

Tsakiraki M, Grammatikopoulou MG, et al. Nutrition transition and health status of Cretan women: evidence from two generations. *Public Health Nutr.* 2011 May;14(5):793-800. Epub 2011 Jan 28.

Willcox DC, Willcox BJ, et al. The Okinawan diet: health implications of a low-calorie, nutrient-dense, antioxidant-rich dietary pattern low in glycemic load. *J Am Coll Nutr.* 2009 Aug;28 Suppl: 500S-516S.

Chapter 8

Archer T, Fredriksson A, et al. Influence of Physical Exercise on Neuroimmunological Functioning and Health: Aging and Stress. *Neurotox Res.* 2011 Jul;20(1):69-83. Epub 2010 Oct 15.

Daley A, Macarthur C, et al. Exercise participation, body mass index, and health-related quality of life in women of menopausal age. *Br J Gen Pract.* 2007 Feb;57(535):130-5.

Daley AJ, Stokes-Lampard HJ, Macarthur C. Exercise to reduce vasomotor and other menopausal symptoms: a review. *Maturitas.* 2009 Jul 20;63(3):176-80. Epub 2009 Mar 13.

Esposito K, Maiorino MI, et al. Determinants of female sexual dysfunction in type 2 diabetes. *Int J Impot Res.* 2010 May-Jun;22(3):179-84. Epub 2010 Apr 8.

Fogelholm M, Kronholm E, et al. Sleep-related disturbances and physical inactivity are independently associated with obesity in adults. *Int J Obes (Lond).* 2007 Nov;31(11):1713-21. Epub 2007 Jun 19.

Gardiner PA, Healy GN, et al. Associations between television viewing time and overall sitting time with the metabolic syndrome in older men and women: the Australian diabetes obesity and lifestyle study. *J Am Geriatr Soc.* 2011 May;59(5):788-96.

Hopps E, Canino B, Caimi G. Effects of exercise on inflammation markers in type 2 diabetic subjects. *Acta Diabetol.* 2011 Mar 24. [Epub ahead of print]

Landmark T, Romundstad P, Associations between recreational exercise and chronic pain in the general population: Evidence from the HUNT 3 study. *Pain.* 2011 May 20. [Epub ahead of print]

Mirzaiinjmabadi K, Anderson D, Barnes M. The relationship between exercise, Body Mass Index and menopausal symptoms in midlife Australian women. *Int J Nurs Pract.* 2006 Feb;12(1):28-34.

Nicholson G, Hall GM. Diabetes mellitus: new drugs for a new epidemic. *Br J Anaesth.* 2011 May 24. [Epub ahead of print]

Puetz TW, Flowers SS, O'Connor PJ. A Randomized Controlled Trial of the Effect of Aerobic Exercise Training on Feelings of Energy and Fatigue in Sedentary Young Adults with Persistent Fatigue. *Psychother Psychosom.* 2008 Feb 14;77(3):167-174 [Epub ahead of print]

Rao MN, Blackwell T, et al. Association between sleep architecture and measures of body composition. *Sleep.* 2009 Apr 1;32(4):483-90.

Sandoo A, van Zanten JJ, et al. The endothelium and its role in regulating vascular tone. *Open Cardiovasc Med J.* 2010 Dec 23;4:302-12.

Seals DR, Jablonski KL, Donato AJ. Aging and vascular endothelial function in humans. *Clin Sci (Lond).* 2011 May;120(9):357-75.

Seals DR, Walker AE, et al. Habitual exercise and vascular ageing. *J Physiol.* 2009 Dec 1;587(Pt 23):5541-9. Epub 2009 Sep 1.

Sonnenschein K, Horváth T, et al. Exercise training improves in vivo endothelial repair capacity of early endothelial progenitor cells in subjects with metabolic syndrome. *Eur J Cardiovasc Prev Rehabil.* 2011 Feb 11. [Epub ahead of print]

Tseng CN, Gau BS, Lou MF. The effectiveness of exercise on improving cognitive function in older people: a systematic review. *J Nurs Res.* 2011 Jun;19(2):119-31.

Watenpaugh DE. The role of sleep dysfunction in physical inactivity and its relationship to obesity. *Curr Sports Med Rep.* 2009 Nov-Dec;8(6):331-8.

Winzer BM, Whiteman DC, Physical activity and cancer prevention: a systematic review of clinical trials. *Cancer Causes Control.* 2011 Jun;22(6):811-26. Epub 2011 Apr 3.

Chapter 9

[No authors listed] Curcuma longa (turmeric). Monograph. _Altern Med Rev._ 2001 Sep;6 Suppl:S62-6.

Cohen M. Environmental toxins and health--the health impact of pesticides. _Aust Fam Physician._ 2007 Dec;36(12):1002-4.

Howitz KT, Bitterman KJ, et al. Small molecule activators of sirtuins extend Saccharomyces cerevisiae lifespan. _Nature._ 2003 Sep 11;425(6954):191-6. Epub 2003 Aug 24.

Jaga K, Dharmani C. Sources of exposure to and public health implications of organophosphate pesticides. _Rev Panam Salud Publica._ 2003 Sep;14(3):171-85.

Jurenka JS. Anti-inflammatory properties of curcumin, a major constituent of Curcuma longa: a review of preclinical and clinical research. _Altern Med Rev._ 2009 Jun;14(2):141-53.

Richter ED, Chuwers P, et al. Health effects from exposure to organophosphate pesticides in workers and residents in Israel. Isr J Med Sci. 1992 Aug-Sep;28(8-9):584-98.

Wood JG, Rogina B, et al. Sirtuin activators mimic caloric restriction and delay ageing in metazoans. _Nature._ 2004 Aug 5;430(7000):686-9. Epub 2004 Jul 14.

Chapter 10

Andon MB, Anderson JW. State of the Art Reviews: The Oatmeal-Cholesterol Connection: 10 Years Later. _American Journal of Lifestyle Medicine._ 2008; Vol. 2, No. 1, 51-57 (2008).

Arterburn LM, Hall EB, Oken H. Distribution, interconversion, and dose response of n-3 fatty acids in humans. _Am J Clin Nutr._ 2006 Jun;83(6 Suppl):1467S-1476S.

Bourre JM. Roles of unsaturated fatty acids (especially omega-3 fatty acids) in the brain at various ages and during ageing. _J Nutr Health Aging._ 2004;8(3):163-74.

Costa LG. Contaminants in fish: risk-benefit considerations. _Arh Hig Rada Toksikol._ 2007 Sep;58(3):367-74.

Hanley DA, Davison KS. Vitamin D insufficiency in North America. _J Nutr._ 2005 Feb;135(2):332-7.

Heaney RP, Holick MF. Why the IOM recommendations for vitamin D are deficient. *J Bone Miner Res.* 2011 Mar;26(3):455-7. doi: 10.1002/jbmr.328.

Holick MF. The vitamin D deficiency pandemic and consequences for nonskeletal health: mechanisms of action. *Mol Aspects Med.* 2008 Dec;29(6):361-8. Epub 2008 Sep 2.

Holick MF. Vitamin D: A D-Lightful Solution for Health. *J Investig Med.* 2011 Mar 16. [Epub ahead of print]

Holick MF. Vitamin D: extraskeletal health. *Endocrinol Metab Clin North Am.* 2010 Jun;39(2):381-400, table of contents.

Johnson DD, Wagner CL, et al. Vitamin D deficiency and insufficiency is common during pregnancy. *Am J Perinatol.* 2011 Jan;28(1):7-12. Epub 2010 Jul 16.

Judd SE, Tangpricha V. Vitamin d therapy and cardiovascular health. *Curr Hypertens Rep.* 2011 Jun;13(3):187-91.

Juraschek SP, Miller ER 3rd, Gelber AC. Effect of oral vitamin C supplementation on serum uric acid: A meta-analysis of randomized controlled trials. *Arthritis Care Res (Hoboken).* 2011 Jun 13. doi: 10.1002/acr.20519. [Epub ahead of print]

King DE, Egan BM, et al. Effect of a High-Fiber Diet vs a Fiber-Supplemented Diet on C-Reactive Protein Level. *Arch Intern Med.* 2007 Mar 12;167(5):502-6.

Magalhães B, Bastos J, Lunet N. Dietary patterns and colorectal cancer: a case-control study from Portugal. *Eur J Cancer Prev.* 2011 May 7. [Epub ahead of print]

Merewood A, Mehta SD, et al. Widespread vitamin D deficiency in urban Massachusetts newborns and their mothers. *Pediatrics.* 2010 Apr;125(4):640-7. Epub 2010 Mar 22.

Myint PK, Luben RN, ey al. Association Between Plasma Vitamin C Concentrations and Blood Pressure in the European Prospective Investigation Into Cancer-Norfolk Population-Based Study. *Hypertension.* 2011 Jul 18. [Epub ahead of print]

Rutter M. Incidence of autism spectrum disorders: changes over time and their meaning. *Acta Paediatr.* 2005 Jan;94(1):2-15.

Simopoulos AP. Human requirement for N-3 polyunsaturated fatty acids. *Poult Sci.* 2000 Jul;79(7):961-70.

Springbett P, Buglass S, Young AR. Photoprotection and vitamin D status. *J Photochem Photobiol B.* 2010 Nov 3;101(2):160-8. Epub 2010 Mar 21.

Zerbo O, Iosif AM, et al. Month of Conception and Risk of Autism. *Epidemiology.* 2011 May 3. [Epub ahead of print]

Chapter 11

Bertelli AA, Das DK. Grapes, wines, resveratrol, and heart health. *J Cardiovasc Pharmacol.* 2009 Dec;54(6):468-76.

Contaldo F, Pasanisi F, Mancini M. Beyond the traditional interpretation of Mediterranean diet. *Nutr Metab Cardiovasc Dis.* 2003 Jun;13(3):117-9.

Egert S, Bosy-Westphal A, et al. Quercetin reduces systolic blood pressure and plasma oxidised low-density lipoprotein concentrations in overweight subjects with a high-cardiovascular disease risk phenotype: a double-blinded, placebo-controlled cross-over study. *Br J Nutr.* 2009 Apr 30:1-10. [Epub ahead of print]

Fulkerson JA, Story M, et al. Family meals: perceptions of benefits and challenges among parents of 8- to 10-year-old children. *J Am Diet Assoc.* 2008 Apr;108(4):706-9.

Gibellini L, Pinti M et al. Quercetin and cancer chemoprevention. *Evid Based Complement Alternat Med.* 2011;2011:591356. Epub 2011 Apr 14.

Haber B. The Mediterranean diet: a view from history. *Am J Clin Nutr.* 1997 Oct;66(4 Suppl):1053S-1057S.

Karamanos B, Thanopoulou A, et al. Nutritional habits in the Mediterranean Basin. The macronutrient composition of diet and its relation with the traditional Mediterranean diet. Multi-centre study of the Mediterranean Group for the Study of Diabetes (MGSD). *Eur J Clin Nutr.* 2002 Oct;56(10):983-91.

Larson NI, Nelson MC, et al. Making time for meals: meal structure and associations with dietary intake in young adults. *J Am Diet Assoc.* 2009 Jan;109(1):72-9.

Mancini M, Stamler J. Diet for preventing cardiovascular diseases: light from Ancel Keys, distinguished centenarian scientist. *Nutr Metab Cardiovasc Dis.* 2004 Feb;14(1):52-7.

Nestle M. Mediterranean diets: historical and research overview. *Am J Clin Nutr.* 1995 Jun;61(6 Suppl):1313S-1320S.

Neumark-Sztainer D, Larson NI, et al. Family meals and adolescents: what have we learned from Project EAT (Eating Among Teens)? *Public Health Nutr.* 2010 Jul;13(7):1113-21. Epub 2010 Feb 10.

Noah A, Truswell AS. There are many Mediterranean diets. *Asia Pac J Clin Nutr.* 2001;10(1):2-9.

Quick BL, Fiese BH, et al. A Formative Evaluation of Shared Family Mealtime for Parents of Toddlers and Young Children. *Health Commun.* 2011 May 18:1-11. [Epub ahead of print]

Chapter 12

Antonogeorgos G, Panagiotakos DB, et al. Understanding the role of depression and anxiety on cardiovascular disease risk, using structural equation modeling; the mediating effect of the Mediterranean diet and physical activity: the ATTICA study. *Ann Epidemiol.* 2012 Sep;22(9):630-7. Epub 2012 Jul 24.

Rogers PJ. A healthy body, a healthy mind: long-term impact of diet on mood and cognitive function. *Proc Nutr Soc.* 2001 Feb;60(1): 135-43.

Sofi F, Cesari F, et al. Adherence to Mediterranean diet and health status: meta-analysis. *BMJ.* 2008 Sep 11;337:a1344.

Torres SJ, Nowson CA. A moderate-sodium DASH-type diet improves mood in postmenopausal women. *Nutrition.* 2012 Sep;28(9):896-900. Epub 2012 Apr 4.

Chapter 13

Buckland G, Mayén AL, et al. Olive oil intake and mortality within the Spanish population (EPIC-Spain). *Am J Clin Nutr.* 2012 Jul;96(1):142-9. Epub 2012 May 30.

Colin A, Reggers J, et al. [Lipids, depression and suicide]. *Encephale.* 2003 Jan-Feb;29(1):49-58.

Covas MI. Olive oil and the cardiovascular system. *Pharmacol Res.* 2007 Mar;55(3):175-86. Epub 2007 Jan 30.

Giraldi G, De Luca d'Alessandro E. Dietary habits in Italy: the importance of the Mediterranean diet. *Ann Ig.* 2012 Jul-Aug;24(4):311-7.

Moreno-Luna R, Muñoz-Hernandez R, et al. Olive Oil Polyphenols Decrease Blood Pressure and Improve Endothelial Function in Young Women with Mild Hypertension. *Am J Hypertens.* 2012 Aug 23.

Perez-Jimenez F, Alvarez de Cienfuegos G, et al. International conference on the healthy effect of virgin olive oil. *Eur J Clin Invest.* 2005 Jul;35(7):421-4.

Psaltopoulou T, Naska A, et al. Olive oil, the Mediterranean diet, and arterial blood pressure: the Greek European Prospective Investigation into Cancer and Nutrition (EPIC) study. *Am J Clin Nutr.* 2004 Oct;80(4):1012-8.

Chapter 14

Ullman A. Pasteur-Koch: Distinctive Ways of Thinking about Infectious Diseases. Aug. 2007. *Microbe* (American Society for Microbiology) 2(8):383-7.

Chapter 15

[No authors listed] Silybin-phosphatidylcholine complex. Monograph. *Altern Med Rev.* 2009 Dec;14(4):385-90.

[No authors listed] Zingiber officinale (ginger). Monograph. *Altern Med Rev.* 2003 Aug;8(3):331-5.

Adlercreutz H. Lignans and human health. *Crit Rev Clin Lab Sci.* 2007;44(5-6):483-525.

Ahmad A, Sakr WA, Rahman KM. Anticancer properties of indole compounds: mechanism of apoptosis induction and role in chemotherapy. *Curr Drug Targets.* 2010 Jun;11(6):652-66.

Allen RR, Carson L, et al. Daily consumption of a dark chocolate containing flavanols and added sterol esters affects cardiovascular risk factors in a normotensive population with elevated cholesterol. *J Nutr.* 2008 Apr;13(4):725-31.

Boschmann M, Thielecke F. The effects of epigallocatechin-3-gallate on thermogenesis and fat oxidation in obese men: a pilot study. *J Am Coll Nutr.* 2007 Aug;26(4):389S-395S.

Burton-Freeman B. Postprandial metabolic events and fruit-derived phenolics: a review of the science. *Br J Nutr.* 2010 Oct;104 Suppl 3:S1-14.

Cavell BE, Syed Alwi SS, et al. Anti-angiogenic effects of dietary isothiocyanates: mechanisms of action and implications for human health. *Biochem Pharmacol.* 2011 Feb 1;81(3):327-36. Epub 2010 Oct 16.

Davis PA, Yokoyama W. Cinnamon intake lowers fasting blood glucose: meta-analysis. *J Med Food.* 2011 Sep;14(9):884-9. Epub 2011 Apr 11.

de Souza MO, Silva M, et al. Diet supplementation with acai (Euterpe oleracea Mart.) pulp improves biomarkers of oxidative stress and the serum lipid profile in rats. *Nutrition.* 2010 Jul-Aug;26(7-8):804-10. Epub 2009 Dec 22.

Gemma C, Vila J, et al. Oxidative Stress and the Aging Brain: From Theory to Prevention. In: Riddle DR, editor. Brain Aging: Models, Methods, and Mechanisms. Boca Raton (FL): CRC Press; 2007. Chapter 15. Frontiers in Neuroscience.

Gruenwald J, Freder J, Armbruester N. Cinnamon and health. *Crit Rev Food Sci Nutr.* 2010 Oct;50(9):822-34.

Howitz KT, Bitterman KJ, et al. Small molecule activators of sirtuins extend Saccharomyces cerevisiae lifespan. *Nature.* 2003 Sep 11;425(6954):191-6. Epub 2003 Aug 24.

Jensen GS, Ager DM, et al. Pain Reduction and Improvement in Range of Motion After Daily Consumption of an Açai (Euterpe oleracea Mart.) Pulp-Fortified Polyphenolic-Rich Fruit and Berry Juice Blend. *J Med Food.* 2011 Jul-Aug;14(7-8):702-11. Epub 2011 Apr 6.

Li H, Xia N, Förstermann U. Cardiovascular effects and molecular targets of resveratrol. *Nitric Oxide.* 2012 Feb 15;26(2):102-10. Epub 2012 Jan 4.

Murata N, Murakami K, et al. Silymarin attenuated the amyloid β plaque burden and improved behavioral abnormalities in an Alzheimer's disease mouse model. *Biosci Biotechnol Biochem.* 2010;74(11):2299-306. Epub 2010 Nov 7.

Raza SS, Khan MM, et al. Silymarin protects neurons from oxidative stress associated damages in focal cerebral ischemia: A behavioral, biochemical and immunohistological study in Wistar rats. *J Neurol Sci.* 2011 Aug 11. [Epub ahead of print]

Suganuma H, Fahey JW, et al. Stimulation of phagocytosis by sulforaphane. *Biochem Biophys Res Commun.* 2011 Feb 4;405(1):146-51. Epub 2011 Jan 8.

Wood JG, Rogina B, et al. Sirtuin activators mimic caloric restriction and delay ageing in metazoans. *Nature.* 2004 Aug 5;430(7000):686-9. Epub 2004 Jul 14.

Yu W, Fu YC, Wang W. Cellular and molecular effects of resveratrol in health and disease. *J Cell Biochem.* 2012 Mar;113(3):752-9.

Yun JM, Jialal I, Devaraj S. Effects of epigallocatechin gallate on regulatory T cell number and function in obese v. lean volunteers. *Br J Nutr.* 2010 Jun;103(12):1771-7. Epub 2010 Feb 23.

Zhang X, Shu XO, et al. Cruciferous vegetable consumption is associated with a reduced risk of total and cardiovascular disease mortality. *Am J Clin Nutr.* 2011 May 18. [Epub ahead of print]